# DR. PREPPER

DR.PREPPER

# DR. PREPPER

## THE DISASTER PREPAREDNESS GUIDE TO HOME REMEDIES

## JEFF GARRETT

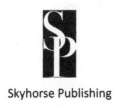

Skyhorse Publishing

10 9 8 7 6 5 4 3 2

Library of Congress Cataloging-in-Publication Data

Names: Garrett, Jeff (Survival and preparedness expert), author.
Title: Dr. Prepper : the disaster preparedness guide to home remedies/ Jeff Garrett.
Description: New York, NY : Skyhorse Publishing, [2016]
Identifiers: LCCN 2016033462 | ISBN 9781510712027 (paperback)
Subjects: LCSH: Emergency medicine. | Survivalism. | Self-care, Health. | BISAC: HEALTH & FITNESS / First Aid. | MEDICAL / Emergency Medicine.
Classification: LCC RC86 .G37 2016 | DDC 616.02/5—dc23
LC record available at https://lccn.loc.gov/2016033462

Cover design by Tom Lau
Cover photo credit: iStockphoto

Print ISBN: 978-1-5107-1202-7
Ebook ISBN: 978-1-5107-1203-4

Printed in the United States of America

# TABLE OF CONTENTS

# I.

# FOUNDATIONS OF SURVIVAL

# INTRODUCTION

Survival preparedness is not to be taken lightly. We live in a society full of comforts, conveniences, and instantaneous answers to all of our questions. We rely on the Internet, 24-hour services, and homogenous one-stop-shop warehouse stores for everything from Q-tips and groceries to electronics and furniture. But what if these things don't last? What if, in an effort to live more independently and explore what nature has to offer, we stumble and can't get help? From a broken down car, to natural disasters and tests of the wilderness, to cyber-attack or infrastructure breakdown, there are threats small and large that everyone should be prepared for. While not everyone has the means and the know-how to ward off institutional threats or the powerful hand of Mother Nature, there is no reason that we all can't arm ourselves with a basic understanding of how to endure, and how to take care of our loved ones in times of threat and disaster, or in the face of wildlife, the elements, and medical emergencies.

Getting yourself out of high-risk situations or knowing what to do when someone goes into shock is not just about having the best supplies or the most experience. These things are undoubtedly essential, but preparedness must first begin on the inside. Maintaining a healthy lifestyle with nourishing foods, regular physical activity, healthy outlets to reduce stress, and regular medical and dental exams are the foundational elements of wellness. Importantly, they can often determine whether or not you can physically endure inclement weather, broken bones in remote places, starvation, stress on the body, wild animal encounters, poisonous plants, and unexpected medical emergencies. Poor diet and sedentary lifestyles can lead to myriad health issues, and the simplest toothache can transform into an abscess that poisons the blood. You never know what small step you could have taken that would have helped you bounce back from an injury or could have reduced your risk of falling ill, so it is important to start preparing for the worst by treating your body the best you can.

This book is a comprehensive guide to knowing a little bit about everything, from what to include when you prepare a survival bug-out-bag, to knowing essential wilderness tips and tricks like water purification and finding shelter, to identifying and treating critter bites and stings or unfortunate brushes with poisonous plants. More importantly, this book provides widespread information on how to cope with medical emergencies, from basic background to home treatment methods for times when hospitals and emergency responders are not within reach. In this book you'll find home remedies and recipes for fundamental treatment options like burn spray and fire ant treatment to stomach-settling teas and anti-inflammatory bone broth. While you never know what's going to happen, this book will give you the resources to plan ahead, assess your situation, find a solution, and help you keep going.

# CHAPTER 1

## YOUR BUG-OUT BAG

### EVERYTHING YOU NEED FOR WHEN DISASTER STRIKES UNEXPECTEDLY

The bug-out bag is a survival essential, but it can mean different things to different people depending on the survival scenario, the length of necessity, the terrain, and the weather. Whether you have a go-to readiness bag for when your car breaks down in a blizzard and you are five miles from home, or you are preparing for something much, much worse, you will need to plan ahead, take stock of the items that are most valuable and will be of the most use to you, and personalize your preparation. While many bug-out bag guides will give you a comprehensive list of hundreds of items to include—from weaponry and portable chainsaws to collapsible tents and fishing supplies—if your time of need is just an overnight in the woods or the wait for a tow truck, then none of these things will be of use to you. Personalization of your bug-out bag is key, so take this into account when putting it together based on your safety, nutritional well-being, overall health, shelter, clothing, and resource needs. If you have a severe allergy or medical condition, make sure to carry any medical bracelets, cards, or information with on or with you at all times. Make your bug-out bag easily customizable, organized, and compartmentalized, so that if you need to grab it but can already tell that you won't be needing that portable saw, your bag is navigable enough that you can just pull it out, save space, reduce weight, and get going.

First aid items are essential for your bug-out bag (BOB), no matter where you are going or what use you think this bag may serve. You will (hopefully) not need all of the items listed, but it is crucial to be prepared and have a sufficient supply of the things that can save your life so that you can keep going until you make it to safety from a hazardous event or location.

## VALUABLES AND INFORMATION

☐ **Flash Drive and Personal Paperwork:** Including but not limited to Social Security cards, passports, driver's licenses, birth certificates, deeds, and financial documents. Scan and save all of your important documents to a flash drive (at least 60GB) and keep it on you at all times.

☐ **E-Reader:** Fancy multimedia and boredom prevention are not the targets here. Products like the no-frills Kindle Paperwhite and Nook have exceptionally long battery lives and can hold literally thousands of texts. You can have survival resources, digital maps, manuals, foreign language dictionaries, and entertainment on hand at a moment's notice, which can make all the difference if you get into a dangerous or unknown situation (or if you just have time to kill).

☐ **Cell Phone, Power Cords, and Chargers:** If you are completely secluded or have limited access to a power source, your cell phone will run out of juice. This doesn't mean you shouldn't prepare, though. Look for items geared for the outdoors, like solar chargers that can be attached to any cell phone. Keep chargers and cords organized and untangled with zip ties and plastic baggies.

## NUTRITION, COMMUNICATION, AND SHELTER

☐ **Water:** Pack as much water as you think you will need and then double it. Of all the survival necessities, water is the absolute last thing you want to go without. You will need it in case of thirst or, exhaustion, and for first aid. If you have to ditch supplies in a dire situation, water goes last.

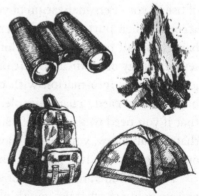

☐ **Lightweight Food:** Get the most out of your packed food items by choosing high calorie, high protein, and high carbohydrate items. Protein bars, trail mix, jerkies, and dehydrated fruits all save on space and offer the most nourishment. Dehydrated meals should be packed for long term survival, but keep in mind that you will need water and cooking tools to rehydrate and cook them.

☐ **Vitamins and Supplements:** If you have limited resources but anticipate a long haul, take daily vitamins and protein supplements to support your nutrition and keep your immune system strong. Vitamin deficiency because of lack of proper nutrition can cause weakness and fatigue and can act as the catalyst to more health complications.

☐ **Solar or Crank Radio:** When you run out of cell phone battery, do not have access to electricity, or you are otherwise stranded, you will want to be able to keep yourself informed.

☐ **Solar or Crank Walkie-Talkie:** Have a two-way radio so you can seek or offer help. Choosing one that doesn't require battery power can help in an emergency.

☐ **Tent, Tarp, and Pack Covering:** Carrying a full-size tent for a family of four can be a hassle, but worth it if you can anticipate your next move, have the ease of vehicular mobility, or do not anticipate a lot of moving around. In the event this is just too much to bear, pack a heavy-duty tarp to serve a number of different needs, from shelter to protecting your wares from the elements. Consider purchasing a covering for your bug-out bag; this can make it more challenging to access the contents of your bag if you need them quickly, but will be useful in protecting your valuables in inclement weather. You can also use a tarp or a heavy-duty trash bag for this same purpose.

☐ **Water-Resistant Bedding:** This is a bit of a luxury, but would be worth it for long journeys or a time when you don't know when your next encounter with civilization will be.

☐ **Quick-Drying Towels:** Easily storable and compact, camping towels are made from microfibers that dry incredibly quickly and can be packed tightly without significantly reducing your bug-out bag real estate.

☐ **Clothing:** Prepare for the elements, with fast-drying materials as your top priority. Include extras of pieces like underwear and socks.

☐ **Handheld and Crank Flashlights:** Flashlights are a must, and depending on your situation, having a crank flashlight can be useful when you have limited access to electricity or if you have run out of batteries.

## TRAUMA KIT

The use of a trauma kit is going to be a matter of life and death. Most first aid kits purchased from pharmacies are under-supplied, containing items like bandages, plastic tweezers, a few pieces of gauze, and a handful small, one-time-use packages of antibacterial ointment or alcohol wipes. These are all important items, but they are really only going to be helpful in minor situations and not if there are multiple large injuries that require repeated care and dressing changes, as may occur if you are out in the wilderness without immediate access to medical care.

- ☐ **Sterile Medical Gloves:** Gloves cannot be emphasized enough. Many sterile plastic gloves are latex, but it is preferable to purchase non-latex gloves, like vinyl, that will pose fewer risks (especially to those with latex allergies) and will be just as useful in an emergency. Never come into contact with blood, open wounds, feces, or other unsanitary or illness-spreading sources without the use of gloves. This will mean the difference between staying safe and contracting a life-threatening infection. At the very least, these items can offer you some peace of mind and reduce any ick-factor. As a last resort, gloves can also help as useful storage devices for fluids, powders, medicine, dry goods, electronics, or anything else that needs to be protected from wet or damp spaces—just tie off the opening like a balloon.
- ☐ **Clotting Powder:** In the event someone has wounds with rapid or excessive bleeding, it will be essential to stop the bleeding immediately. Large, open wounds, arterial hemorrhages, or individuals who are taking blood thinners can face challenges with blood coagulation, so clotting powder like Celox or QuikClot can help close the wound as a complement to other first aid and trauma care. Products like Celox work by pouring the powder into the wound and packing it to form a makeshift stopper plug, but can also be removed for further wound care if necessary. You will want a clotting powder that does not generate heat to reduce the risk of thermal burns to the skin and tissue. Be careful when using clotting powder in windy environments so that excess powder cannot be blown into sensitive places like the eyes and cause damage. Clotting powder is lightweight and usually comes in

small packs that are easily storable. It should only be used in emergency situations, and you should always follow the directions listed on the original packaging, as some clotting powders function differently from others and may have specific warnings for safety of use.

☐ **Iodine, Alcohol, and Antibacterial Wipes or Ointment:** These cleansing and sanitizing items are vitally important to help prevent the spread of infection. Particularly when treating and dressing a wound, you will need to clean the affected area and protect it from potential complications. Iodine has many uses, including the purification of water, so it may be worth it to bring an entire bottle of iodine rather than individual packets that will run out more quickly. Gauge your expectations of how dire the situation you are entering is when packing these items. Is your supply bag just something you are toting with you on a casual hike on a temperate summer day? Or are you going off the grid without a clear timeline for your safe return? If it's the former, you can probably downsize and bring just enough of these cleaning agents while you wait for emergency responders to reach you.

☐ **Gauze, Bandages, and Medical Tape:** Because they are essential for wound care, make sure to have an ample supply of these important items. Your selections should range in size to anticipate any given situation—from minor blisters and cuts to large, unstable wounds. Have a roll of medical tape to help tape up wounds but also as a useful tool for other unforeseen problems, like fixing broken tarps and holding together broken essentials for when you need them most.

☐ **Surgical Stapler and Suture Kits:** Most surgical stapler kits come preloaded with staples and are packaged with a staple remover. Suture kits have several tools, including forceps, hemostats, tweezers, and sterile scalpel blades. When you are in rough terrain or remote areas where severe injury is more likely to occur, these kits can be a matter of life and death. They are generally compact enough that having them in your bug-out bag will not mean foregoing a lot of space. They are not meant for the faint of heart; both stapling and suturing wounds are messy business and should be done with great care. Do not store either of these kits haphazardly—the sharp blades must be kept clean and stowed safely.

☐ **Prescription Medicine:** Include backups of any prescription medication that you or your family members require. If your insurance will allow it, have a full month's supply or more in the event of a disaster that makes obtaining prescriptions difficult or near impossible. If you have an illness that requires injections, like insulin, make sure to bring enough supplies to keep you going.

☐ **EpiPen:** Epinephrine always has a place in a long term bug-out bag. Anyone who suffers from serious allergies will already have at least one on hand, but it is always a good idea to carry one in case someone you come into contact with experiences anaphylactic shock, or if you are confronted with a serious event or medical emergency that induces anaphylaxis. While EpiPens require a prescription, many doctors feel comfortable prescribing them as backups when patients request them.

## Alternative Uses for Tampons

Feminine hygiene in survival situations is incredibly important, and it is easy to take the availability of tampons and sanitary napkins in developed countries for granted. They are both sterile and disposable, which is an advancement that has hugely transformed women's health. In many poor countries, women who don't have access to commercialized sanitary napkins and tampons are relegated to reusing rags during menstruation, which can lead to infection and sometimes death. Although tampons are a necessary item for women when out in the wilderness or in areas where access to a pharmacy may be sparse, there are also many other helpful ways to use tampons when you are stuck in a bind or have a surplus of these helpful products.

### First Aid

Tampons are sterile wads of cotton, which means that they can be used reliably as a bandage. Whether you have to plug up a gushing wound or nosebleed, or you are working with a larger wound or abrasion, they are the perfect, travel-friendly first aid tools in a pinch. For wounds with a large surface area, simply break apart the cotton to get more from material to help cover the wound and create a bandage. You can use the sterile tampon string to tie off the bandage, as well.

### Water Purification

Tampon cotton can be used to soak up sediments and other things lingering in a water source when you need the water for drinking or cooking. This method will *not* purify the water or remove harmful bacteria, but it can help get rid of nasty particles before you plan to boil or otherwise purify the water. Simply cut off the bottom of a water bottle, plug up the spout with the tampon cotton, and turn spout-side-down before pouring water through it. For the most effective route to cleaner water, create a small hole in the cap and keep the cap on so that the water does not gush through the cotton and spill.

### Storage

Tampon wrappers are usually plastic cylinders, which means that a number of different small items can be kept safely away from the elements. If you don't have a dry place to put matches, store them in the tampon wrapper and tie off the end with the tampon string. Just be careful when opening the plastic so as not to tear all the way down the length of the wrapper.

## HEALTH, HYGIENE, AND COMFORT SUPPLIES

☐ **Personal Hygiene:** A bar of soap and roll of toilet paper will pretty much cover all the bases, but if you have room, include other personal hygiene products like baby wipes, Q-tips, shampoo, and hand sanitizer. Baby wipes are a fantastic way to keep clean when you do not expect to have access to a shower, so put this high on your list of priorities. Hand sanitizer is never your *best* option as compared with regular soap and warm water (since it can kill good bacteria in addition to the bad), but sometimes when you're faced with seriously unpleasant circumstances a squirt from a bottle of hand sanitizer will be your savior.

☐ **Dental Hygiene:** This should probably go without saying, but oral hygiene is still vitally important, even if you are off the grid or will be otherwise away from your home base for an extended period of time. Complications of tooth decay, abscesses, mouth infections, cold sores, canker sores, toothaches, broken or lost teeth, and other serious oral ailments need to be cared for as much as any other part of your body. Include a portable toothbrush, toothpaste, floss, and numbing gels for oral wounds and aches (like Anbesol) to take care of your mouth.

☐ **Feminine Care:** Your medical supplies should include tampons or sanitary napkins to manage menstruation. This is not a luxury; this is a necessity. Improper management of menstruation, like repeated or extended use of the same tampons, sanitary napkins, or rags can cause toxic shock syndrome, infection, or something more deadly. Whether you are traveling with women or not, you should always have these items on hand in the event you come across someone who needs them. There are many compact tampon designs—some with applicators and some without—that make storing and traveling with tampons a lot more convenient. Feminine products are sterile when coming straight from the packaging, and can therefore also be used as an alternative forms of medical supplies. Take a look at the sidebar on page 10 for more information on alternative uses for feminine products.

☐ **Condoms:** No need to skirt around the issue: condoms are absolutely necessary in any long-term survival scenario. If you are off the grid or away from most of civilization, you will already have enough to deal with to survive, and adding pregnancy, HIV, and other STDs to the list would only make matters exponentially more complicated and dangerous. Like feminine hygiene products, condoms also serve a number of different purposes in addition to prophylaxis. Take a look at the sidebar on pages 14-17 for more information.

☐ **Pain Relievers:** Include acetaminophen (Tylenol), aspirin, and ibuprofen (Motrin or Advil) in your kit for pain relief. Acetaminophen helps reduce fever and pain, and should be taken according to package instructions, as misuse and taking more than the recommended dose can cause serious medical problems or death. Ibuprofen is an NSAID (nonsteroidal anti-inflammatory drug) that helps reduce fever, pain, and inflammation. Aspirin is also an NSAID, but has more significant blood-thinning effects, which is why it is often prescribed to individuals at risk for blood clots and heart attack. It is not recommended to take any of these medicines with alcohol.

☐ **Respiratory Medicines:** Antihistamines, allergy medications, and decongestants should have a space in your bug-out bag medicine cabinet. In the event you come down with a head cold brought on by cold or damp weather, environmental factors, or if you have an allergic reaction, you should not be relegated to just toughing it out.

☐ **Stomach Illness:** Whether you accidentally ingest contaminated drinking water or experience food poisoning, you will need anti-diarrheal medicine like Pepto-Bismol or Imodium, antacids like Tums or Rolaids, and mild laxatives to alleviate any unpleasant stomach illness symptoms. Particularly when you are in an isolated area, extreme temperatures, or if you do not have access to water, diarrhea can be life-threatening. Include a packet of oral rehydration salts to help with potential dehydration from stomach illness.

☐ **Sunscreen and Sunburn Treatment:** Sunny, cloudy, cold, or hot—no matter the climate, UV rays will still reach you. Pack SPF 30 sunscreen to protect your skin, especially your face, from the elements. Skin damage, sunburns, sun blisters, and sun poisoning are the last thing you need when out on your own, so protect yourself accordingly. Severe complications of sun exposure can be horrifyingly painful, debilitating, and exhausting. Always take precautions with sun exposure, and in the event of sunburn, include cooling gels like aloe vera or comfort creams containing camphor, aloe, or menthol to help soothe your skin.

☐ **Other Medical Needs:** Consider carrying other medicines that will ease any potential discomfort, such as sleep aids like melatonin, cough drops, and motion sickness medication. These are more circumstantial, and you will need to determine whether or not they are worth the space in your first aid kit.

☐ **Bug and Insect Repellent:** This needs no introduction, because any interaction with biting or stinging insects will only cause problems for you wherever you are. Make sure to bring DEET-based repellents for optimal protection, as well as mosquito netting to protect you while you sleep or traverse muggy, swampy, or otherwise insect-infested areas.

☐ **Backup Corrective Lenses:** If you wear corrective lenses or contacts, have an extra pair of glasses or set of contacts (with cleaning solution and commercial saline solution). Glasses are at risk for breaking and contact lenses are very difficult to keep up if you do not have modern conveniences available. If you prefer contacts, make sure to properly clean and store them with sterile cleaning solution.

☐ **Comfort-Related Items:** Items like hand warmers, cooling packs, ChapStick or other lip balm, and unscented and alcohol-free body lotion can all make your life a lot easier in extreme conditions. Particularly when your skin is cracked or peeling from harsh cold or heat, it is important to avoid products containing alcohol. Scented lotions generally contain alcohol, which can be painful to use on cracked or sensitive skin.

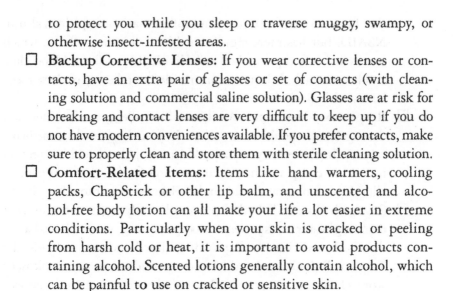

## Alternative Uses for Condoms

Packing condoms in your bug-out bag or stow-away first aid kit may not be your first thought, but when the going gets rough, they should actually be a top priority. In addition to preventing pregnancy and the spread of STDs, which are both hugely important in a worst-case-scenario survival situation, there are several different ways that condoms can get you out of a bind and safeguard even more of your prized possessions. Keep in mind that all of these suggestions are for unlubricated latex condoms, particularly for food and water storage. Most drug stores tend to carry lubricated condoms, so you may need to do some hunting online to stock up. Condoms are very elastic and can be stretched a surprising amount, but they are also prone to tearing. For any super-sensitive storage, make sure to protect the condom with a sock or clothing to prevent something from popping or tearing it. For anything that needs to be opened quickly without potentially damaging the contents, always tie off the condom around something small and sturdy, like a pencil, piece of wood, toggle, etc. This will allow you to undo the knot more easily so that you can potentially reuse the condom (not for pregnancy or STD prevention, however), as well as prevent any spillage from liquid contents like water.

### Protecting Your Valuables

True to their original intention, condoms can protect more than just physical valuables. Use unlubricated condoms to keep electronics like cell phones, chargers, powder cords, and even batteries dry. Condoms are very elastic, meaning that they can hold a surprisingly large amount of objects that you'd prefer to keep dry. While you *can* stuff many of your belongings into one condom, it is probably better to disperse these into multiple small bundles so you don't need to worry about breakage.

### Water and Food Storage

Condoms can hold up to a gallon of water—one gallon! This makes condoms one of the most space-saving food storage receptacles out there, particularly if you are in a situation where you have lost or broken existing water bottles, if you can't carry more with you, or if you just want to downsize. While this isn't the best method to carry food and water, because it's not foolproof, it can help you out in a pinch. As mentioned earlier, after you have filled the condom with water or food, tie it off with a toggle—essentially anything small and stick-like that will allow you to tie and untie the ends with greater ease. Be careful when pouring liquid into the condom, as it is prone to breakage. Do so by setting the bottom down on a surface (rather than holding it in the air while you transport the liquid). Because condoms—particularly ones that are being stretched—can break incredibly easily, whether it's a brush from a pinprick or a blade of grass. To prevent breaking, tearing, or leaking, protect the condom by keeping it stored in a sock or article of clothing. You should still purify your water after storing it in a condom.

### First Aid

Unlubricated condoms are the mittens of the rubber glove world. When you don't have latex or vinyl gloves to use to perform first aid, use your trusty condoms. Insert your hand into the condom

*(Continued on next page)*

and gently work on the area of concern. This will help prevent both you and the victim from potential infection from exposure to open wounds, sores, blood, and bodily fluids. In the rare event that you will need to use a tourniquet, condoms are stretchy enough that they can be used to tie off the area without causing too much damage to the skin and muscle tissue surrounding the area.

## Inclement Weather

Heavy downpours, snowstorms, and wading through bodies of water can be problematic if you have limited clean, dry clothing available. When you can anticipate these events, protect your dry clothing with condoms. Wear unlubricated condoms over your dry socks to keep the socks from soaking. If you are wearing thin gloves that are not water-resistant and can soak easily, wear the condoms over those, too! You may feel silly, but being clean and dry in a survival scenario—whether it's long term or you're unsure how long you will be forced to brave a cold rainstorm—can prevent anything from minor discomfort to debilitating problems like frostbite, hypothermia, and infection.

## Fire Starters

The ability to start a fire in a survival scenario is crucial, which means that it is just as important to keep matches, tinder, and kindling protected from the elements. Stuff these into a condom to prevent them from getting wet or damp so that you can use them when you need them most. Latex condoms are also highly flammable, so while they are not ideal environmentally, they can help get a fire going. Keep a little bit of tinder inside the condom when lighting it to lengthen the amount of time the flame keeps going. When you don't have matches or lighters available, you can also use a condom to create downward pressure when starting a fire the old-fashioned way. When starting a fire with a traditional spindle, hearth board, and a bearing block, make a loop on each end of the condom for each of your thumbs. Insert your thumbs into the thumb loops, and stretch the center of the condom over the spindle. As you get the spindle moving with your hands, the elasticity from the condom will create downward pressure on the spindle for better friction, while also keeping it in place. You can also fill the condom with water and treat it as a magnifying glass for sunny-day fire starting.

*Pillows, Flotation, and Rope*

While condoms can act as a multipurpose tool for so many crucial tasks—from carrying water and first aid to starting fires—there are a few more handy uses that can be helpful when you're low on supplies. To make small pillows, stuff condoms with soft grass, leaves, or cattail fluff. Blown-up condoms can work as fishing bobbers or low-burden flotation devices. You can even use the stretchy condoms to set up a slingshot when hunting in the woods, or to use as a replacement for rope when tying up a tent or other structure.

## OTHER PRACTICAL TOOLS AND SUPPLIES

- ☐ **Swiss Army Knife or Multiuse Tool**: The original survival necessity, having a multiuse tool on hand can help you out of all sorts of tricky situations. Of course, these tools aren't just about cutting through cords, opening bottles, or clipping off that pesky hangnail. Heavy-duty multiuse tools will have pliers, screwdrivers, and sturdy knives that can be handy in a number of unforeseen circumstances. These can be fairly high in price, but the cost is worth it for something so multifunctional and compact.
- ☐ **Hunting Knife**: Have a sturdy, sharp, slightly serrated knife for any number of uses, whether it's hunting and food preparation, protection, or an everyday tool to get you through the difficulties of tough terrain or malfunctioning equipment.
- ☐ **Wine Key/Cork Screw**: Many multiuse tools will already have a corkscrew, but in case yours doesn't, have one on hand for food and beverage needs. Compact, restaurant-quality wine keys, which have small blades to slice through foil, are helpful for box cutting and have a number of additional uses other than just opening up a bottle of Bordeaux.
- ☐ **Cooking and Eating Utensils**: Some multiuse tools will have eating utensils attached, but if not, you can also purchase

camping equipment for this purpose. Collapsible bowls are extremely useful.

☐ **Sewing Kit:** Most local pharmacies sell sewing kits that take up almost no space in a secondary pocket or compartment of a bag. If even this is too much room, just keep a spool of thread and a needle on hand in the event of wardrobe or equipment malfunction.

☐ **Rope or Paracord:** Rope will do, but paracord is better. Paracord is incredibly strong and can be used for hunting, fishing, setting up shelter, hiking, traversing difficult territory, survival, and dozens of other uses. Paracord does not rot or mildew, so the integrity of the cord will last significantly longer than many ropes that can soak-through and weaken.

☐ **Twist Ties:** From closing up food items and keeping power cords organized and separate, twist ties are infinitely useful. And, they take up almost no room.

☐ **Heavy-Duty Plastic Bags:** Waste disposal, storage, shelter, waterproofing, warmth, you name it—you will have a use for plastic bags, and when you do, you will want them to be strong.

☐ **Compass:** Not everyone will need a compass, but it never hurts to have one. Particularly if you are packing your bug-out bag for excursions in the wilderness, this will be an important part of your journey.

☐ **Matches and Lighters:** This should be obvious, but double up on matches and lighters. Have them at the ready and make sure they are kept properly stored in dry and waterproof spaces. Consider purchasing steel and flint fire starters (the size of a set of keys) from a hardware store. You will need them.

☐ **Fire Starters:** Whether you have a plastic baggie filled with dryer lint or you purchase fire sticks or fire starting pellets from an outdoorsman or hardware store, make sure you have these at the ready. Keep them sealed in plastic baggies or special compartments so that they do not get damp from the elements.

☐ **Trick Candles:** More than just a party trick, trick candles can be incredibly useful when starting a fire in an environment with high winds. Since they continue to light and relight, you will not waste more matches than you need on getting your fire going. You can put them out by soaking them in water.

☐ **Water Filters or Water Purification Tools:** See the section on water purification on page 29. This will be essential if you are in even a moderate survival scenario. Humans needs at least 2 quarts (8 cups) of water per day to survive, and if your only water source is unpurified or even the tiniest bit questionable, you can make your situation a whole lot worse.

☐ **Plastic Baggies:** Use small sandwich and freezer bags to organize the contents of your bug-out bag. Throwing everything into your pack will make dire situations where you need to think and act quickly even more challenging, so it is a good idea to separate the essentials into organized, logical groups that you can pull from at a moment's notice. Many backpacking stores will have special bag organizers for purchase, but plastic baggies are inexpensive, efficient, and can be labeled easily.

## *Chlorination*

Purifying water with bleach will work well, but it is a very precise process that needs to be done carefully to avoid poisoning yourself or contaminating your water supply. Do not use special bleaches that are color-safe, scented, or combined with other cleaners; ones that have been sitting on a shelf longer than a year; previously opened bottles; or products that are otherwise distinct from traditional bleach. Make sure to read the label of the regular bleach, and look for the note that says that it contains no more than 8.25 percent sodium hypochlorite. The amount of bleach you add to the water will depend on the amount you are purifying—adding too much bleach will become problematic. Use a sanitized medicine dropper to distribute the bleach, following the table below.

| Volume of Water | Amount of Bleach to Add* |
|---|---|
| 1 quart/liter | 2 drops |
| 1 gallon | 6 drops |
| 2 gallons | 12 drops (1/8 teaspoon) |
| 4 gallons | 1/4 teaspoon |
| 8 gallons | 1/2 teaspoon |

*http://water.epa.gov/drink/emerprep/emergencydisinfection.cfm.

# CHAPTER 2

## HOW TO LAY THE GROUNDWORK

### BASIC HOW-TOS FOR KEEPING THINGS
### FROM FALLING APART

First aid and home remedies are not just about knowing how to stitch up wounds, brew healing tonics, and mix soothing salves. Prevention, preparedness, cleanliness, and a little bit of know-how are the dividing line between you and a nasty infection, broken bone, or debilitating ailment. From building shelter to purifying water to starting a campfire, this chapter will delve into the many pivotal steps you should take in a survival scenario. Whether your electricity is out from a storm, you get lost on a hike, or you have been forced to go completely off the grid because of a nationwide disaster, these foundational methods of survival and self-reliance are your best defense.

## How to Build Shelter

Shelter can mean a lot of different things to different people. Depending on the severity of your survival situation—short-term where you only have to stay warm for a night, or something more long-term—there are several different ways to build reliable shelter that will keep you warm, dry, and able to get going the next day. Whatever your situation may be, the first and most important step in seeking shelter is to analyze your surroundings. Particularly in cases of extreme cold or heat, building shelter and finding water are crucial to ensuring your safety or the safety of your loved ones. Find or set up your shelter in areas near fresh water, but not so close that you are sharing space with water-hovering insects like mosquitos or are in danger of flooding. Take into account that dry riverbeds or trails can be perfect paths for flash flooding if severe weather hits, so even this poses a risk. If you are in the woods or near a cliffside, stay clear of dead trees or loose rocks, as these pose a real risk of falling and harming you and your shelter.

When choosing the kind of shelter you plan to build, take account of the environment around you, how long you will be there, and any potential changes in weather. Do you need to build a fire inside the shelter because it is too cold, windy, or rainy outside? In that case, you would need a structure that vents the smoke while also insulating the heat. When setting up a space inside your shelter for sleeping, make sure to put protective space between you and the ground. Especially during frigid weather, the cold ground can absorb body heat and make it harder to stay warm as the night progresses. Place dry brush like leaves, sticks, and evergreen boughs to form a six-inch-thick layer over the area you will use for sleeping and cover it with a tarp, blanket, or sleeping bag if you have them available. Ideal camping sites are on a slight downward incline so that rain will not pool around you. In cases where extreme weather may cause flooding in your shelter, dig a trench around the area for easier drainage. In the opposite situation of desert heat, it is a good idea to set up your shelter out of direct sunlight; remain wary of how much sun the shelter is getting during the day, as temperatures can increase so intensely that your new home is now an oven. Since it is unlikely that you will happen across a fully stocked log cabin for your convenience in a survival scenario, this list of shelters will help you get by—whether you just need to camp out for a few hours, or build something a little longer term.

## Tents and Hammocks

While this section will go into more depth about do-it-yourself shelters, it is worth noting that camping tents and hammocks are well worth the purchase if you can afford them. While large four-person tents can be difficult to carry if you have to stay on the move, they will make your life a lot easier if you don't have to go too far and are experiencing wind and cold. Many tents have vestibule compatibility, which can be helpful in keeping out rain, drying clothes, and protecting your belongings that would not otherwise fit in the tent. When carrying a large tent is just too much, try tenting hammocks. Hammocks made from parachute material are water-resistant and easy to string up between trees, and a simple tarp hung above the hammock can protect you from the elements. If you can splurge, some hammocks are designed specifically as suspension tents.

## Tarps, Parachutes, and Plastic Sheeting

In any survival scenario, having tarp, poncho, or parachute material with you can be a lifesaver. It can protect you from wind, cold, and extreme heat, while also blocking out pests, insects, snakes, and other potential nuisances or hazards. In situations when you cannot build a closed-in shelter and there will be open air, just make sure to position the material so that it blocks the direction of the wind, sun, or precipitation.

## Securing a Tarp or Plastic Shelter

Regardless of the shelter you are setting up with this material, you should be mindful of how you secure it to the ground so that it can last for many uses, if not indefinitely. If you are using basic plastic sheeting or a tarp *without* grommets (the metal rings that allow you to feed rope through them), you should avoid securing the base of your shelter with stakes or any other method that will tear holes in the material. This will compromise the shelter and cause leaks. Instead, place rocks, bags of sand, logs, or any other heavy objects along the base of the material to keep out the elements.

In the event your tarp or parachute material does have grommets, you can secure the base of the structure by using aluminum poles, camping stakes, or paracord. Your ropes or paracords should always be several feet longer than the tent you plan to build. If you are using paracord, it can be helpful to feed the cord through the grommet from the bottom-up and then wrap the cord around a wooden stick. Thread the other end of the cord back through the grommet and then secure it to another stake or object to dig into the ground. This will help prevent tearing of the grommet and tarp in the event of tugging or aggressive winds.

## A-Frame Tent

This tent is the most straightforward tent you can build using a tarp, plastic sheeting, or parachute material. It looks like a simple pup tent and can be built with paracord or even ski poles. Find a location where you can secure two ends of the tent—preferably between two trees (or the two ski poles) about six to ten feet apart. If the tarp has grommets, feed the paracord through them on each end of the tarp when making the peak; this will help keep the tarp in place so it doesn't shift or become lopsided with wind or movement. Tie the paracord between the two trees, securing the knots tightly. If your tarp does not have grommets, it is best to secure the base with heavy rocks so that the tarp does not tear from puncturing it. Otherwise, use stakes, paracord, or other objects you have on-hand that will keep the base snug to the ground.

## Tarp Teepee

Teepees are regarded as one of the best wilderness shelters for a reason. They are relatively easy to construct and keep the warmth in. This version of a teepee does not require the framework of a traditional one. With the help of a low-hanging branch, simply gather material from either end of the tarp, wrap it tightly into a nub with cord, and tie the remaining cord to the branch. The rest of the tarp will hang down, and from here you can spread the material to make the teepee shape and secure the base to the ground using rocks or logs. Alternatively, you can throw the rope over the branch and wrap it around the tree for a pulley-like system that lets you raise and lower the tent. Make sure you have arranged it so that there is an opening to get in and out of the shelter. The higher you pitch the teepee, the better it will be at shedding water, snow, and wind. A shallow pitch will be less effective at reflecting water, but will offer more room inside.

## Tarp Lean-To

Lean-tos are simple in design, but pretty effective at blocking out the elements if you construct them against another surface like a cliff, incline, or densely situated trees. In this scenario, simply spread the tarp out until it is completely flat, and tie the top left and right ends to trees. Secure the base of the tarp with stakes or paracord (if your tarp has grommets), or with heavy rocks and logs. This shelter is not meant for long-term use, but it will work if you are in a bind and need to get out of the rain and cold.

## One-Man Hut

When you are on your own, need protection from the cold, and are short on tools and building supplies, this shelter can make a big difference. Find a long, sturdy tree limb between six and ten feet long, depending on your height. One end of the limb will rest on the ground, and the other should rest two to three feet in the air against a stable structure, like a rock wall or a stump, or over a tripod made of branches that are snugly buried into the ground. With the center pole in place, begin by gathering branches of varying lengths to align vertically along the length of the center pole. The more branches you can find to lean against the center pole, the more insulated and stronger the structure will be. When each side of the pole has a line of branches and limbs, gather dry brush like leaves, grass, small sticks, and evergreen branches to cover the walls. Build this section out until it is thick (at least a couple of feet in width) to ensure that wind and rain will be effectively blocked. If there is snow on the ground, use the snow to help insulate as well.

## Snow Cave

In the event of a snowstorm or blizzard, finding shelter is top priority. The best way to build a safe snow cave is to start by finding areas where the work is already done for you: find a snowdrift or hillside area that has a lot of snow cover. Be wary of choosing a snowdrift that is in an area prone to avalanches or that have snowdrifts set higher on the hillside than yours—the higher snowdrift could give way and destroy or envelop the one you are in. If you are able to find a snowdrift, make sure it is at least five feet high. You can use this as your foundation to build a safe shelter that will hold in a lot of warmth.

Building a snow shelter is not about speed. Exerting a lot of effort and sweating can be dangerous—this will lead to loss of energy and a drop in body temperature. Move at an easy pace and take breaks. If you are starting from scratch and not from a snowdrift, take your time while shoveling snow to make a large mound that is at least five feet high. Make sure to stomp or roll on the snow to make it more compact as you set it in place. Light and powdery snow does not set easily, so give it time to set and become compact as you work to ensure a stable structure; this can take several hours. Once your snow cave is at least five feet high, allow it to set for at least two hours. From there, place two ski poles or large sticks about twelve to eighteen inches into the center of the dome at about two feet apart, like flags. These will be your point of reference when you are digging out the inside of the cave.

It is safer to build a snow shelter with a partner. He or she should be equipped with a shovel and stand outside of the cave as you dig in the event of collapse. When digging out the snow cave, start by digging a small trench at the doorway so that the threshold is constructed lower than the inside of the cave. This will help maintain heat inside. Continue by shoveling out a tunnel from the center of the snow mound. Shovel from this central tunnel only until you have cleared at least two feet, and then you can begin to hollow out the cave. When you can fit your whole body in, continue scraping out the dome. If you clear enough snow that the bottoms of the ski poles are exposed, you have reached your stopping point for the ceiling. The roof should be at least one foot thick, and the walls should be at least two feet thick.

With enough snow, consider carving out benches to sleep on or shelves for storage. The benches will help you stay warm by elevating you off the ground. Layer the floor with insulation, like evergreen or fir boughs, sticks, sleeping bags, or blankets, to help contain the heat and prevent it from being absorbed by the ground. Create one-inch ventilation holes by inserting a ski pole, or stick at an angle through the ceiling and clearing a small airway. If it feels like too much warm air is escaping, you can block the holes with clothing or a snowball. Just make sure to remove the blocker and keep the air hole clear when going to sleep or if the air gets stuffy. Smooth out any bumpy snow on the inside of the dome so that a change in temperature won't cause the jagged parts to drip. If the temperature is below freezing and you have extra water, pour the water over the outside of your snow shelter to help harden the surface and set the structure. DO NOT do this if the air is above freezing, as it will melt the snow and weaken the integrity of the snow cave.

Place bright markers on the outside of the snow cave so that other people (if they should cross paths with you) do not accidentally damage the pile. Use clothing or backpacks as your door so that animals and cold air do not come in. Store shovels inside the cave in the event of ceiling collapse or avalanche so that you can dig yourself out.

## How to Dispose of Human Waste

Disposing of solid human waste, while not the most desirable of tasks, is critically important in order to remain healthy and take care of the environment around you. Most people produce two to three pints of urine and one pound of solid waste per day, which means it can add up quickly if you no longer have access to running water and functioning toilets.

There are a few situations that will require you to dispose of solid waste in more creative ways, some of which are limited to the home, others when you are out in the wilderness or in rural areas. Those in urban areas have some convenient options, but truth be told, if there is a long-term crisis that interrupts water flow and sewage draining, you may actually be better off in rural areas.

## Disposal at Home

If you are still able to maintain your residence but do not have running water, you will need to get a little crafty. If you have a septic system, you are one of the lucky ones. Septic systems do not rely on public water for flushing, so you will still be able to flush your toilet, assuming you are using your water sparingly. In this situation, it is best to be conservative with how often you flush and what you choose to put down the drain. Allow few uses for liquid waste and save your flushes for solid waste instead. Use toilet paper sparingly, and wrap up and throw away feminine products or wet wipes rather than flush them down the toilet. You do not want to risk clogs or backup, as this can have a snowball effect, create many other problems, and potentially contaminate your fresh water.

If your home is connected to the public sewer system and you no longer have running water (or if the reserve water from your septic system is no longer available), you can still flush your toilet. The easiest option is to pour a bucket of water down the toilet, which triggers a syphoning action that will automatically flush the toilet for you. Anyone who regularly pours the gray water from washing his or her floors down the toilet will have already witnessed this time and time again. Never use drinking water to flush the toilet. This is a waste of a perfectly good resource; instead, use water that you have already used for cleaning (like gray water from dishes or floor washing) or collected rainwater. You can also add water to the cistern, or the back tank of the toilet. Add enough so that the water reaches the float, at which point you will be able to flush.

## Indoor Latrine

If using precious water—even dirty old sink water—is no longer an option in your home, you can create a makeshift latrine out of your existing toilet. Place a heavy duty, double-lined plastic bag into the bowl of the toilet. Close the toilet seat over the bag so that it stays in place. Use this latrine for solid waste, and then cover each contribution with wood ash, kitty litter, sawdust, quick lime, or dirt. (Limiting this latrine to solid waste is helpful in reducing smell—while solid waste can certainly have an unpleasant odor, urine is what tends to intensify these odors until your bathroom starts to smell like a porta potty.) When the bag is about two-thirds full, add some disinfectant or a dirt and chlorine mixture, and then store the bag until you can dispose of it. You can also use this same method with a five-gallon plastic bucket if you cannot, or prefer not, to use your toilet. It is helpful to put a couple of two-by-fours on the edges of the bucket for seating, or you can even purchase toilet seats that are specially designed to fit on such buckets. Keeping the bathroom area clean and the latrine closed-off when not in use is very important; if insects, flies, pets, or pests get into the waste and then find themselves in other parts of your home or food supply, the bacteria can spread and potentially cause illness.

## Outdoor Disposal

Outdoor waste disposal is fairly easy, albeit sometimes messy, but still requires some wherewithal, cleanliness, and attention. Contamination with water sources and living environments is a very real issue: exposure to human waste can affect water and food supply, crops, and sanitation. Waste disposal outside generally requires some excavation. You will need to find appropriate areas to dig a hole or trench, which absolutely *must* be at least fifty to two hundred feet away from water supplies, such as lakes or rivers, from paths or highly-trafficked areas, and from shelter. Even if a location is not near any of these things, make sure it isn't an area that has the potential for water flow when it rains (downhill trails, runoff, or drainage areas, etc.). Locations that see a lot of sunlight are especially useful for waste disposal, as the heat and light dry out the soil more quickly, leading to more efficient decomposition. In the outdoors, never use wet wipes or other synthetic sanitary napkins that cannot biodegrade or that you cannot properly throw away. Use toilet paper sparingly, and if need be, use rocks or non-prickly, non-poisonous leaves to clean yourself. If you are unable to wash your hands afterward, be extremely careful about using leaves as a replacement for toilet paper. Leaves can tear, which can soil your hands with hazardous bacteria.

## Cat Holes

Cat holes are your best option in a short-term scenario. With a trowel or another digging tool, create a hole that is about eight inches deep and four to eight inches in diameter for your solid waste. Dispose of your used toilet paper in the same hole, and then fill the hole back in with the removed dirt. You can make several of these in the same area, though just be careful that you clean up after yourself and have covered the holes properly. If you are still in the same location over the next few days, the hole or holes may appear sunken from the soil settling, so you can add more dirt to the top to even out the ground.

## Outdoor Trench Latrine

When you are not just passing through a given area and need to make a toilet that will last a bit longer, you can build a multiuse, makeshift trench. A trench will require more thoughtful excavation and planning to ensure that the hole will be clear from foot traffic and be safely away from water sources or crops in the event of flooding or severe weather. Just as with cat holes or other outdoor toilets, the trench should be dug at least fifty to two hundred feet away from water sources, trails, or shelter. Dig the hole so that it is at least one foot wide and two feet deep. If you anticipate more than a week or so of use, consider digging it several feet deeper or be prepared to scout multiple locations. If you have wood available, set up a border around the trench so that the hole is closed off, or you can place boards down if you prefer to sit rather than squat. After each use, cover the waste with about an inch of wood ash, dirt, sawdust, kitty litter, or the like. You can dispose of toilet paper in these holes, but make sure to use as little as possible, and use non-bleached, recycled toilet paper if possible. When the trench is not in use, cover it with a board or mark it very visibly so that no one will accidentally step in it.

Taking care of human waste does not have to be a challenge. Make smart choices when deciding disposal locations, and always be mindful to clean up after yourself. If done properly, anyone who happens to come across your path after you have been there will be none the wiser that you just made the area your own personal rest stop.

## HOW TO PURIFY WATER

When water is in limited supply, there are several steps you can take to find or purify water. If you are still in your home but you no longer have running water, you have a few options before you no longer have any drinkable water. This section will cover these, and then move on to how to purify water when you do not have modern conveniences available to you, whether because your home infrastructure has been compromised and all of your available water has been consumed, or if you are out in the wilderness and must make do with what is available.

Humans can survive without food for a long time, but $H_2O$ is another story. Even in the most disastrous of situations in which you are rationing everything, you must drink at least two quarts (eight cups) of water to survive per day. Carbonated beverages like soda or beer will dehydrate you; do not use them as replacements for proper hydration. It is better to delay eating food than to delay drinking water—never ration water less than you need to survive in the hopes that you will come across more later, because you will be risking your life. When water is low and you are unsure of the next time you will find some, try to stay cool and limit your physical activity to prevent perspiration.

## Take Advantage of Existing Drinking Water

If you no longer have drinking water stocked up and must take desperate measures before you can reassess your situation, most homes will be equipped with at least a few options for a last-resort. Start by locating the potable water sources in and around your home. Water found in fish tanks, toilets, heating systems like hot water boilers or radiators, swimming pools, hot tubs, waterbeds, puddles, or standing water are all **unsafe** to consume. Even if your water is turned off or is no longer running, it is still possible to extract healthy drinking water from the pipes. Force air into the pipes by turning the faucet on to its highest capacity until you can see some water drip out. Go to the faucet that is at the lowest point in your home (e.g., the first floor or basement sink, if you have one), place a receptacle underneath, and turn it on to retrieve what you can.

You can also drink the water that drains from your water heater in your home, but keep in mind that you should only attempt draining the water from the heater if the gas or electricity in your home is turned off. If it hasn't, turn it off so that you can drain the water without jeopardizing any of the heating systems in your home. Open the drain at the bottom of your hot water tank and let it pour into a bucket or other receptacle. Make sure the hot water faucet is on, but the water intake valve is off. If the problem gets resolved and the running water supply is restored to your home, make sure that you refill the water tank before turning the gas or electricity back on. Seek the assistance of a professional to turn the gas back on, as doing so incorrectly can be hazardous.

When these resources have been exhausted, keep in mind that certain foods like watermelon, celery, and cucumbers all have high water content and can help keep you hydrated in a dire situation. Canned foods like vegetables and fruit are stored in water, as well. Drink these to help stay hydrated, or melt the ice cubes from your freezer. It is unlikely that you will be able to find enough of these items to replace an entire day's worth of water (let alone for multiple people), but they are good resources in the event that you have limited options and need to make do while you seek alternatives.

## Water Treatments and Purification

If you reach the point where you no longer have fresh, potable water available to you, there are a few different ways to purify water that you would have otherwise avoided drinking. Lake and river water; cloudy, colored, or standing water; and other similar sources are all examples of water that needs to be purified before you can drink it. Contaminated water, often caused by exposure to human or animal fecal waste, can cause severe gastrointestinal illness like diarrhea, cramps, and vomiting. While this may sound like a passing inconvenience, in a survival scenario, they can cause severe dehydration, which can become life-threatening.

Unless you feel like carrying around a Brita pitcher everywhere you go, methods like filtering, boiling, adding chlorine, and distilling can all help to purify the water you are working with. While these methods are not perfect, some of them can be combined for healthier drinking water and improved flavor. Chlorinating water or adding iodine alone will not necessarily prevent the aforementioned gastrointestinal discomforts or other illnesses, but combining it with filtration can. Keep in mind that boiling water, chlorination, and distillation will all kill microbes and make the water safe to drink, but only distillation will remove contaminants like chemicals, salt, and heavy metals. Water should be treated and purified any time you need to drink, brush your teeth, make ice, wash dishes, prepare food, and any other situation in which you may be rinsing with water and somehow ingesting it later.

## Filtering

Filtering water is an important first step before boiling or otherwise purifying the water you are going to use, especially if you do not have access to chemical cleaners. Particularly if your water source is visibly cloudy, darkly colored, or is from a questionable source, you will want to start by creating a makeshift filter. If you have coffee filters, clean cloths, or paper towels on hand, they will work well. Let the water settle, and then pour the water through the clean filter. You may want to repeat this process with clean filters once or twice before moving on to the boiling process.

If you are in an outdoors scenario where the conveniences of coffee filters are unavailable to you, another useful filtration method starts with a water bottle and ends with some rocks and sand. Cut the bottom off of a water bottle, and then turn it over so that the cap is facing down. Secure the bottle in this position so that it will not be able to move when you pour water through it. This next part will be a little bit like making a bottle of multicolored sand art at a county fair. Except with this bottle, you are going to create several layers of filters within the bottle to help catch the existing impurities in the water between the layers before the water pours from the tap at the bottom. The first layer closest to the cap will be made of pebbles, followed by a layer of sand, a piece of cloth like cheesecloth or clean bandages, charcoal, another layer of cloth, another layer of sand, and finally another layer of pebbles. Each of these layers works together to remove the impurities, particularly the charcoal, which is often used in natural medicine to remove toxins from the body. Pour the water through this filter, being careful not to spill, and allow it to pour into a receptacle or container. Once the water is filtered, you will still need to boil it to kill any remaining bacteria or viruses.

## Boiling

Boiling is a tried and true method of sanitizing water, and while it is the simplest way to get rid of any leftover impurities, it is also the most fail-safe of all of the techniques available. Unlike chemical purification, there is no opportunity to measure chlorine incorrectly and risk harming yourself, let alone drinking chemical-flavored water that is anything but refreshing. Most importantly, boiling water kills viruses, protozoa, and pathogenic bacteria that are present in unpurified water and it helps reduce the risk of getting ill. In a large stove pot, bring the water to a rolling boil for a minimum of one minute. For higher elevations (5,000 feet or 1,000 meters above sea level), you should boil the water for at least three minutes. Water will evaporate during this process, so if you start with a gallon of water, do not expect to come away with a gallon of water. Once the water has boiled for several minutes and purified, allow it to cool on its own to room temperature. You can then store the water in sanitized containers or water bottles. Boiled water is not always the best-tasting water, but oxygenating it can help improve the quality a bit. To do this, transfer the water back and forth from one container to another, or add a pinch of salt per liter of water you store.

## Distillation

Distillation is the only process that will truly remove all harmful germs from your drinking water. As a result, it is slightly more complicated and requires more patience than the alternative methods of water purification. The distillation process is similar to boiling, but in this case, you will be collecting the vapor that results from the boiling process and using that as your safe water source. Repeat the same filtration steps to remove all of the larger impurities like grit and dirt. If the water is cloudy, allow it to settle. Pour water into a large stockpot. Tie a cup to the handles of the lid so that the cup hangs down in the pot when the lid is in place. The cup should sit right side up and there should be enough room between the top of the cup and the underside of the lid so that water can drip down. When the water boils, the steam will collect on the underside of the lid and then drip into the cup. When the cup is full, pour the water into a clean container. Let the water cool to room temperature and then cover the container before storing. Repeat this process until you have the desired amount of purified water.

## Chlorination

Purifying water with bleach will work well, but it is a very precise process that needs to be done carefully to avoid poisoning yourself or contaminating your water supply. Do not use special bleaches that are color-safe, scented, or combined with other cleaners; ones that have been sitting on a shelf longer than a year; previously opened bottles; or products that are otherwise distinct from traditional bleach. Make sure to read the label of the regular bleach, and look for the note that says that it contains no more than 8.25 percent sodium hypochlorite. The amount of bleach you add to the water will depend on the amount you are purifying—adding too much bleach will become problematic. Use a sanitized medicine dropper to distribute the bleach, following the table below.

| Volume of Water | Amount of Bleach to Add* |
| --- | --- |
| 1 quart/liter | 2 drops |
| 1 gallon | 6 drops |
| 2 gallons | 12 drops (1/8 teaspoon) |
| 4 gallons | 1/4 teaspoon |
| 8 gallons | 1/2 teaspoon |

*http://water.epa.gov/drink/emerprep/emergencydisinfection.cfm.

If your bleach contains 5.25 percent to 6 percent sodium hypochlorite, you can adjust your measurements. In this circumstance, you can add eight to nine drops to one gallon of water. Once you have added the bleach to the water, let the water rest for thirty minutes. After it has settled, there should be a light chlorine odor, but not overpowering. Add more bleach by repeating the first step if you cannot smell the chlorine, but be careful not to overdo it. If there is a strong chlorine flavor, let the water sit for several hours. If there is still a strong flavor so much that it burns or stings, you have used too much bleach.

### Iodine

Iodine has long been used as a disinfecting agent for wounds, surgery, and water purification. As with chlorination, it is helpful to start by filtering out all of the larger impurities with a coffee filter or water bottle filter. For every quart or liter of water that you intend to disinfect, add five drops of 2 percent tincture of iodine. Increase this amount to ten drops if the water is particularly cloudy or discolored. Gently mix in the iodine and then let the mixture stand for at least thirty minutes before drinking.

### Granular Calcium Hypochlorite (HTH)

HTH is a powerful oxidant that must be handled and stored very carefully. The cleansing process of HTH is effective in the same way as chlorinating water, but in this case, you are adding an extra step by preparing the bleach solution from its granular form. When making this solution, do so in a well-ventilated area and protect your eyes and face with goggles, glasses, gloves, and a mask. Combine a heaping tablespoon or ¼ of an ounce of HTH with two gallons of water and stir until thoroughly dissolved. Once your chlorine solution is ready, you will use one part of the chlorine solution for every 100 parts of water, as seen in the conversions below. The measurements provided are best for when you are disinfecting large quantities of water, rather than a simple vessel of drinking water.

| Volume of Solution | Volume of Water |
|---|---|
| Half Cup (4oz.) | 3 ⅛ gallons |
| Cup (8oz.) | 6 ¼ gallons |
| Pint (16oz.) | 12 ½ gallons |
| Quart/Liter (32oz.) | 26 gallons |

### Water Purifying Tablets

There are many different types of water disinfection tablets that are geared toward the hiking and camping community. These will come in handy, and the packaging will provide appropriate instructions for the proper dosing of a given brand. You can find such tablets online and through adventure, hunting, or camping retailers.

## Maintaining Proper Hygiene

It should go without saying that good hygiene is one of the most effective methods of warding off illness, preventing the contamination of drinking water or food supply, and staying generally healthy. Be sure to wash your hands with soap and water after going to the bathroom or after coming into contact with bodily fluids and animal waste. You do not need to use hot water for hand washing to be effective, but do scrub with soap for at least twenty seconds before rinsing. Unless you are in a pinch, regular hand soap is preferable to hand sanitizer, as sanitizer tends to dry the skin and is literally overkill—it will kill even the good bacteria on your skin, leaving room for bad bacteria to flourish later.

## How to Store Food

Always think ahead and stockpile long-lasting foods, like canned, dried, or airtight meats, fruits, vegetables, and grains. Keep them in a cool, dry place and make sure they are properly labeled by item and date. Store seeds, bulbs, and other crop starters in airtight and dry containers as well. Freezing food items will be helpful if you expect to have electricity, but for disaster preparedness, you are better off with dry storage and anything that can be moved without the change in environment drastically affecting the quality of the food. Home canning, tightly sealed mason jars, airtight containers, and plastic bags are all effective methods of long-term food storage.

### Keeping Food and Fluids Cool

If you are in a high-heat climate, be it in the desert or just on a scorching summer day in the mountains, you will need to keep your beverages and any perishables you may have cool. While it is not recommended to go trekking into high heat with fresh fruits, veggies, and meats packed away in your bag, there may come a time, such as after hunting, when you need to store food in a cooler climate for a short period of time. If you are near a body of water, like a river, the easiest way to keep things cool is to pretend you planned on going lobstering. If you have water bottles, sealed food items, or even cans of beer, all you have to do is put them in an egg crate, trap, or even a heavy-duty garbage bag, tie it to a sturdy rope, and then anchor that rope on land. (If you use an egg crate, make sure you have found a way to cover the top or place it in an area without a strong current.) Cool mountain streams will be just the right temperature to keep everything crisp.

If you are not located near a body of water, you can dig a hole in the ground that is the height of the container. This method is best utilized in a shady area with cool, damp soil to help maintain lower temperatures. If you are in a desert, dig an open hole and lay a tarp over the top for shade.

### Dehydrating Food

Dehydration does wonders for the longevity of meats, fruits, vegetables, and herbs. Dehydration helps extend the shelf life of food and maintain essential vitamins and nutrition that can be lost in other forms, but it also helps condense precious space when mobility is one of your highest priorities. It is important that any foods that you dry out at home are done so thoroughly so that you do not risk the food spoiling. Make sure to store your dried foods in airtight containers until you plan to use them. Dehydrated food can be rehydrated before it is consumed, which makes for cooking good stews over a campfire. Using a store-bought food dehydrator is easiest, but in the event that you do not have access to electricity or simply can't carry around a giant appliance, you have options.

Typical garden herbs like rosemary and lavender are the easiest to dehydrate. Simply tie them together in bunches and hang from a string, door frame, or beam in a cool, dry location. Allow them to dry out for a couple of days, or until they crumble to the touch.

Leafy greens, vegetables, and fruits are the next step up in complexity, but even these are easy to dehydrate even in the most rugged of scenarios. Cut larger fruits and vegetables into small, thin slices. Poke holes, pit, or cut berries in half for the best exposure to heat and air. Spread these out on a large, clean screen and leave the screen in direct sunlight, or set them over a low fire until they are thoroughly dried.

Dehydrating meat and fish is still quite easy, but you run more of a risk of the meat going rancid or not drying out completely if the process is not done properly. As with fruits and vegetables, cut the meat into small pieces, and make sure it is sliced very thinly. Remove any excess fat, as this is much more difficult to dry out and poses the risk of going bad. The key is to give the meat as much exposure to air as possible. Season the meat with salt and set over a low fire until the meat is tough and dry.

## How to Start a Fire

Fires can mean the difference between life and death. Whether you are trying to keep warm or are cooking food, it is essential to know how to start a fire when you are on your own or away from modern conveniences, heat, or cooking methods. If you do not have matches or lighters, you will need to know how to start one with your own hands and the resources you have available.

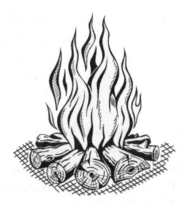

*A variation of a crisscross-style fire.*

## Setting Up a Campfire

Start by gathering all of the materials you will need for a fire. These include tinder, kindling, firewood, and matches or a lighter if you have them. Tinder is your base ingredient, and as such it is instrumental in getting your fire started. Wood shavings, wax, dryer lint, or strips of paper and cardboard all function as tinder. Kindling is a little bit bigger, usually in the form of small, dry twigs and branches. Evergreen branches are great kindling because they catch fire easily and the resin is flammable. This is what makes the crackling and popping noise that you may have heard if you have ever used evergreens in a campfire. Firewood should be properly dried out before using.

Prepare a clear, safe location to start your fire. Make sure it is away from things that can easily catch fire, like dry brush and leaves, clothing, or your shelter (if the fire you are starting is inside your shelter, just be careful to keep the fire contained). There should be about eight to ten feet of space between your fire pit and anything flammable. If you are using a campsite that has already had a fire, make sure to clear the excess ash and any leftover pieces by moving them to the edge of the fire pit or circle, or by shoveling the contents out. You can use the ash later to put the fire out.

Use rocks to line the edges of the fire pit so that you protect yourself and the fire from spreading. In the center of your fire pit, make an even pile with the tinder that is about a foot in diameter. This will be the base of your fire, and should be equidistant from the firewall.

37

For a teepee-style campfire, start by arranging the small kindling into a teepee shape at the center of the fire pit (on top of the tinder). Repeat this process with the firewood so that you have one teepee inside the other. Carefully light the fire from the kindling until the flames spread to the firewood. You may need to blow lightly on the embers until the flames catch.

When building a more traditional crisscross campfire, simply crisscross your kindling over the tinder, and then the crisscross your firewood over the kindling. Light the kindling and watch it carefully until the fire catches the firewood. The crisscross shape is conducive to long-lasting campfires that can stay lit and warm for several hours.

## How Start a Fire When You Don't Have Matches

Always try to have matches or a lighter on you, because starting from scratch is a challenge, dependent on the items you have available to you, and exhausting. You can use a lens, make sparks with steel and flint over tinder, or use the friction method. Make use of the tools you have around you to help the process along, and always keep your fire starters dry.

There are a few different ways you can start a fire without matches or a lighter, and the one that requires the least exertion is probably the old magnifying glass route. You may not have a magnifying glass on you, but anything with a lens, like eyeglasses or binoculars, can do the trick. Clean the lens and then angle it beneath the sun and at about a 30-degree angle from the tinder and kindling that you are trying to ignite. Adding a couple of drops of water can help hone the sunlight to be a more direct beam. It may take a few minutes, but you should start to see smoke. Work quickly and allow the tinder to catch with the kindling. No magnifying glass or pair of glasses? Get a condom. This sounds strange, but it can work: fill the condom with clear water and use it in the same way that you would a magnifying glass.

With a steel and flint, you use the flint or other piece of rough, sharp stone to strike the steel to create sparks. Do this directly over your tinder, and once the tinder catches fire, you can add it to your kindling.

Starting a fire using friction methods is the most challenging and will take a bit of sweat, but it will get a fire going. You will need a piece of fireboard, a spindle (which can be a dry branch), and a bed of tinder or fire starter. On the edge of your fireboard, cut a V-shaped hole out of the wood and carve out a depression right next to it. Place a piece of bark underneath the V, and place your tinder over the depression. You will scoop the burning embers onto the bark to transfer to your kindling. Stand or kneel over the fireboard to keep it steady and place the spindle in the depression. With two hands, start spinning the spindle rapidly to create friction.

If you can make a bow, this will drastically decrease the amount of energy you expend trying to start a fire with just your hands and the spindle. Make a bow out of a bendable branch, about two feet long and attach a sturdy rope to either end. Keep the rope or cord just loose enough so that you can twist the rope around the spindle. Using a socket (e.g., a piece of rock that has a small depression or space for the top of the spindle to fit), keep the spindle steady, and run the bow back and forth across the spindle so that the base turns rapidly. The socket will allow the spindle to keep spinning without harming your hands. Do this quickly and repeatedly until you start to see embers in the tinder. Once there are embers, brush them onto a piece of bark or directly onto kindling to get the fire going.

## How to Make a Splint

While chapter 7 will delve into fracture and wound care further, you should have basic knowledge of making a splint in an emergency situation. When you are in a setting requiring this kind of medical attention, time will be of the essence to reduce pain and begin administering first aid. A splint is generally necessary in the case of a fracture (broken bone) or a severe wound that can be come aggravated if it is moved. The splint immobilizes the body part to prevent further damage while you are en route to medical help or while you wait for emergency care to come to you.

In the case of a fracture, which can occur with only a slight break in the bone, a jagged break, or a clean one, you will need to make a splint to help minimize pain and to stabilize the injured body part. Particularly in the cases of open fractures, when the bone has torn through soft tissue, you should start by cleansing, treating, and bandaging the wound. Assess the injured limb for healthy circulation, as sometimes grossly bent fractures can put pressure on or pinch your veins and interrupt normal blood flow. Do this by comparing the affected area to the area beyond the fracture or to another body part (if an arm is broken, compare it to the other arm).

Once you have treated any wounds and assessed the circulation, you can move on to immobilizing the injured limb. It is not a good idea to move the injured bone in order to make the splint. Generally speaking, you should splint the body part in the position in which you found it while you wait for a medical professional to care for it. If you believe that you will not be able to reach medical care for an extended period of time and the body part is severely misaligned or bent, or if it is evident that circulation is being compromised, then you can—very gently—move the limb back to its normal position. Do not twist or jerk the limb as you do this.

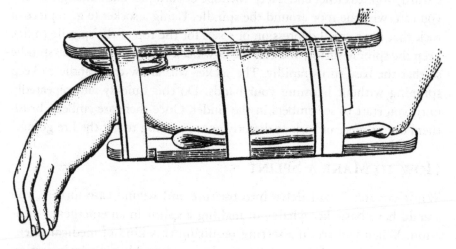

*A splint supporting an arm.*

You can make a splint with many different items. Use what is available to you, but straight boards, sticks, rolled up newspaper, ski poles, or any other rigid item can function well as splints. The item you use should be longer than the affected area so that it will remain in place and there is no risk of further damage. When making the splint, be sure to include the joint above or below the affected area to secure the position of the splint properly and prevent further damage. If you are dealing with a fracture of the forearm, for example, you should also secure your wrist and elbow in the splint, because these joints are connected to the affected area. Place padding in between the rigid piece of the splint and the injured limb. You can use clothing, padding from a backpack or camping equipment, egg crates, or any other soft item you have on hand that will act as a cushion.

Secure the injured bone or bones to the splint with tape or ties. You can use neckties, bandanas, shoelaces, belts, clothing, rope, and any other similar items in order to do this. Do not secure the ties directly over the fracture or the wound; instead, tie it off at either end of the splint. Be careful not to secure the splint too tightly; you do not want to cut off circulation. For fingers and toes, you can use the neighboring bones as a splint. Simply tape the broken finger or broken toe to the one next to it to help stabilize it, but be careful not to tape it too tightly. Lightly wrap more cushioning around the splint if you are at risk of bumping it or injuring it further.

Monitor the splint to make sure that it there is no increased swelling, numbness, and paleness. If the pain increases significantly from having made the splint, undo it immediately and reassess the situation, as you may have splinted the injured bone incorrectly. Seek medical attention if you can. Allowing the injured body part to go untreated—particularly in the cases of open fractures—can leave you vulnerable to infection and improper or crooked healing.

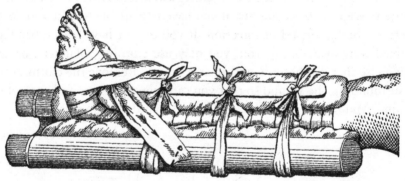

*A leg splint made of found items.*

## Splint Basics

- Clean and treat the wound
- Assess circulation
- Place light padding in between the injury and the item you use for the splint
- Use rigid items like a board, stick, or neighboring appendage to stabilize and restrain the bone

(Continued on next page)

- Secure the splint with tape or ties on either side of the break, but not directly over it
- Do not tie the splint too tightly
- Monitor the injury and the splint over time
- Seek medical attention

## How to Make a Tourniquet

In the event of severe and uncontrollable blood loss, you may need to use a tourniquet to stop the bleeding. Improperly executed tourniquets, or ones that have been left on for too long, can cause muscle and tissue death. This can result in the loss of a limb, so applying a tourniquet should not be taken lightly and should only be done in extreme scenarios. Tourniquets should only ever be used on limbs like arms and legs, and never around the neck. Whenever you are dealing with rapid blood loss, it is important to put pressure on the wound and stop the bleeding before or while you call for emergency medical attention. Always choose sterile gauze to stop the bleeding first if you have it available so that you do not increase the likelihood of infection. If you do not have sterile bandages immediately available to you, you may use clothing, blankets, or anything else that is otherwise within arm's reach. Remove the clothing that is surrounding the wound so that you can properly assess and control the wound. You may need to tear or rip it off in order to do this.

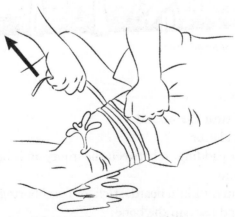

*A tourniquet without a a torsion device.*

To make the tourniquet, you can use flexible material like bandages, clothing, a necktie, a bicycle inner tube, a luggage strap, a bandana, etc. Do not use paracord or other forms of rope, as this material is not flexible enough and can cause tissue damage. You will also need a torsion device to tighten the material around the wound, which can be anything rigid like a stick. Wrap the limb about two inches above the wound on the side closer to the heart and tie in an overhand knot. Wrapping the wound below blood flow to the heart will be ineffective. Also make sure not to wrap the tourniquet around a joint. Place the stick or makeshift torsion device above your overhand knot. Tie another knot above the stick to secure it. Twist the stick in one direction until the tourniquet tightens enough to stop the bleeding. From here, use the remaining material to tie the torsion device to the tourniquet, keeping everything in place.

The tourniquet is not a long-term solution to blood loss. Lack of blood flow to limbs can cause tissue death, so you will need to seek emergency medical attention to treat the injury if at all possible. When you think the bleeding has stopped, usually after an hour or so, assess the wound and see if you can release the tourniquet. If blood continues to flow, replace the tourniquet and bandages until you can properly control the bleeding. Treat the victim for shock while you wait for professional medical attention.

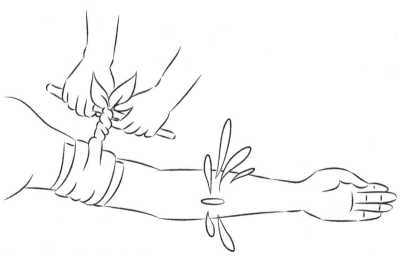

*A tourniquet using a torsion device.*

## Tourniquet Basics

- Stop the bleeding with sterile gauze or clothing
- Remove excess clothing
- Tie off the wound with flexible material
- Do not tie over a joint
- Tie at least two inches away from the wound and closer to the heart
- Place a torsion device on top of the overhand knot, then tie another knot to secure
- Turn the torsion device in the same direction until the tourniquet is tight
- Secure the torsion device and the tourniquet so it does not come undone
- Monitor the bleeding and treat the victim for shock

# CHAPTER 3

## THE HOMEMADE APOTHECARY

### NATURAL RECIPES FOR HOMEMADE SALVES, TEAS, AND TREATMENTS

### HEADACHE REMEDIES

Whether you are a chronic migraine sufferer or only get headaches every once in a while, they can be debilitating, sabotage productivity and movement, and are often difficult to alleviate. In the event of a migraine, make sure to reduce, avoid, or get rid of all potential aggravators: lower or turn off any harsh lights (or wear sunglasses), do not consume alcohol, stay hydrated with cool water, eat regularly to stay nourished, and place a cool compress or ice pack on the area where the pain is the most severe. Do not ice the skin directly—make sure to have a towel or cloth in between your skin and the ice pack to avoid tissue damage. Ice on and off every fifteen minutes. When cloistering yourself in a dark room with an ice pack on your head just isn't doing the trick or when you have run out of pain relievers or prefer not to use them, here are a few natural home remedies to help break up some of that searing pain.

### Lavender Oil

Lavender oil is often credited with headache and migraine relief. While it is not to be consumed orally, it does not have to be diluted like many other oils used for medicinal purposes. Place a drop or two on your fingertips and rub on the temples and wrists. The heat from your wrists will bring out the aroma of the lavender more quickly. Place your hands on your temples so you can breathe in the lavender oil for a soothing way to ease your migraine. Alternatively, you can make a lavender steam with lavender oil and inhale the steam for headache relief.

*Lavender Steam Recipe*
*Ingredients*

3–4 cups water
2–4 drops lavender oil

*Method*

Boil the water. Add 2–4 drops of lavender oil to the boiling water in a bowl. Placing a warm, damp towel over your head and the steaming bowl, then breathe in the steam from the lavender to help reduce the pain of your headache or migraine. Be careful not to get too close to the steam so as not to burn your skin.

## Peppermint Oil

Similar to lavender oil, peppermint oil is often hailed as a migraine treatment. Peppermint has been shown to help stimulate blood flow and open up the sinuses. Drinking peppermint tea can be a soothing way to calm a difficult tension headache. If you prefer something a little more direct, rub peppermint oil on the temples to help break up your headache and fuel circulation.

## Feverfew

Feverfew is a member of the daisy family, and when taken in capsule, whole leaf, or tea form, it can help prevent and calm migraine symptoms. When taking feverfew capsules, make sure to follow the directions and take the recommended dose provided on the bottle—usually no more than two 250-milligram pills per day. Alternatively, you can eat about three small feverfew leaves, or steep fresh or dried feverfew in a tea.

*Feverfew Tea Recipe*
*Ingredients*

2 cups water
2 tablespoons feverfew, fresh or dried

*Method*

Boil 2 cups of water. Place 2 tablespoons fresh or dried feverfew leaves in a tea steeper. Drop the steeper into the boiling water and let steep for

8–10 minutes. If you do not have a tea steeper, just add the leaves in whole and then strain them from the hot water before drinking. The feverfew brew will be very bitter, so you may want to sweeten it with honey.

## STOMACH TROUBLES

Nausea, diarrhea, constipation, and other stomach discomforts can be a big challenge, but there are a handful of natural remedies to help alleviate these pains to keep you healthy, happy, and energetic. Many natural remedies for headaches, like peppermint and steam aromatherapy, can also soothe upset stomachs. Pure peppermint oil can be too strong for some, particularly those with stomach ailments, so try using a peppermint steam or drinking peppermint tea to reduce discomfort. (For the peppermint steam, follow the directions for lavender steam and use peppermint oil, starting with 2 drops of peppermint oil, increasing the amount if desired.) When stomach-related issues arise, be sure to stay hydrated with clean drinking water and avoid soda and alcohol, which will both cause dehydration.

## CONSTIPATION REMEDIES

### Coffee

Most coffee drinkers are familiar with this, but drinking a few cups of coffee in the morning wakes up your digestive system as much as it boosts your energy. Drink one to two cups of coffee to help with constipation, but it's best to stop there. Too much coffee can actually have the reverse effect and cause constipation and dehydration.

### Blackstrap Molasses

While over-the-counter laxatives or a couple cups of coffee will always do the trick, there are natural alternatives to alleviate constipation if you prefer the natural route or if you can't reach a pharmacy. This sticky sweetener is a stool softener and can help move things along when constipation becomes an issue. Take 2 tablespoons of blackstrap molasses directly. Keep in mind that molasses is incredibly thick, sticky, and sweet (think of a dog eating peanut butter), so you can dilute the blackstrap molasses with water to make it more drinkable.

### Blackstrap Molasses Recipe
*Ingredients*

2 tablespoons blackstrap molasses
2 cups water (optional)

*Method*

Boil the water. Stir the molasses into the hot water until it is dissolves, and then drink the mixture once it has cooled a bit.

## Olive Oil

Olive oil can help alleviate constipation by jumpstarting your digestive tract. Take olive oil in the morning before breakfast and wait for it to work its magic. Since drinking olive oil is not the most appetizing of morning drinks, mix it with lemon juice to make for a tastier option.

### Olive Oil Recipe
*Ingredients*

½ lemon
1 teaspoon olive oil

*Method*

Juice the lemon, removing the seeds. Whisk the lemon juice and olive oil together until evenly blended. Drink prior to eating.

## NAUSEA AND UPSET STOMACH REMEDIES
### Ginger

There is a reason why ginger ale is any grandmother's go-to cure for an upset stomach. Ginger can help improve circulation, reduces inflammation, and helps soothe the intestinal tract so that symptoms associated with stomach flu, such as nausea, vomiting, diarrhea, and stomach cramps.

*Ginger Tea Recipe*
*Ingredients*

1 tablespoon (about 1 inch) fresh ginger
2 cups boiling water
juice of ½ lemon
1 teaspoon honey

*Method*

Make homemade ginger tea by peeling 1 inch of fresh ginger. Grate the ginger, or slice it thinly and add to 2 cups boiling water. Let the ginger steep for 10 minutes. Strain out the ginger pieces and add the juice of ½ lemon and 1 teaspoon of honey to sweeten.

## COLD AND FLU SYMPTOM REMEDIES

When cold and flu-like illnesses strike, they hit hard. Colds are the tropical storm to the flu's hurricane—both feel pretty terrible, but the flu is far worse and can come with severe complications, so it's important to take them seriously. While the two are not one and the same, the symptoms are often similar. Congestion, sneezing, sore throat, and achiness are all incredibly unpleasant, so you should have a few home remedies in your back pocket to help you or your family members get through them.

To make your life a little bit easier, here are a few natural options for bolstering your immune system and taking care of some of these nasty symptoms. Make sure to stay hydrated and get plenty of rest while suffering from a cold or the flu, and to seek medical attention.

## Bone Broth

Chicken soup may very well be the oldest of cold and flu remedies, and for good reason. The collagen found in beef, poultry, pork, and even fish broth have immunity-boosting properties that help alleviate inflammation, settle the stomach, and provide nourishment to get you back on your feet. Choose bones from organic, grass-fed animals and select parts that have a significant amount of bone marrow, fat, and connective tissue, like knucklebones, joints, and oxtail. This recipe has the option to include vegetables and spices, but because you will be cooking the bones at such a high temperature or for many hours, these ingredients will be boiled to death and not offer all that much in the way of flavor. Consider using them when making a soup with the broth, or add them at the very end of the process.

When dealing with symptoms of a cold or influenza, be sure to drink several cups of bone broth daily. Prepare the bone broth and use it for drinking, and any leftovers can be incorporated with cooking, whether that means making a nice pot of chicken soup, or using it to flavor vegetables on the stove.

### Bone Broth Recipe
*Ingredients*

5 pounds beef, pork, or poultry bones
5 quarts water (**6 quarts if using optional ingredients)
2 tablespoons apple cider vinegar
2 tablespoons salt

*Optional Ingredients:*

2 celery stalks, cut into 2-inch pieces
2 carrots, cut into 2-inch pieces
1 large onion, quartered
1 head garlic, peeled
2 tablespoons whole peppercorns
**increase the water content by 1 quart if adding optional ingredients

*Method*

Add all of the bones (and optional ingredients, if using) to a stockpot, slow cooker, or pressure cooker. Add the water, apple cider vinegar, and salt. Cover and bring to a boil. Lower the heat to a simmer and cook for 12–24 hours on the stovetop, 24–48 hours in a slow cooker, or 3 hours in a pressure cooker. Never leave the stovetop unattended.

## Apple Cider Vinegar for Sore Throats

Apple cider vinegar has seemingly endless uses, from cooking and cleaning, to settling the stomach, whitening teeth, and boosting energy. When suffering from a sore throat, the acidity in a little apple cider vinegar can help flush out nasty cold-related germs. Taking it straight can be difficult to swallow, literally, so you may want to dilute it with water.

*Apple Cider Vinegar Recipe*
*Ingredients*

¼ cup apple cider vinegar
¼ cup warm water

*Method*

Combine the apple cider vinegar and warm water. Use as a gargle. Repeat every few hours while sore throat symptoms last.

## Homemade Vapor Rub

There are few things more comforting when you have chest congestion than applying some smooth, minty vapor rub to the skin. The soothing balm opens up your sinuses upon inhalation and seems to be just the refreshing, calming effect you need. The main ingredients here are a carrier (base) oil like extra virgin olive oil, almond oil, or coconut oil; beeswax; and anywhere from 40–60 drops of aromatic essential oils. You can play with these by mixing and matching, but be careful—the scents can be overpowering. If making the vapor rub for children or babies, reduce the essential oils by half so that the vapor rub is not overwhelming, and use sparingly. Check with a pediatrician before using vapor rub on children.

### Ingredients

½ cup extra virgin olive oil (or other carrier oil)
2 tablespoons beeswax pellets
10–20 drops eucalyptus oil
10–20 drops peppermint oil
5–10 drops rosemary oil
5–10 drops of another aromatic oil, like lavender (optional)

### Method

Using a double boiler on low heat, heat the carrier oil and beeswax until just melted. (If you do not have a double boiler, you can put them in a heat-safe container like a mason jar, place the jar in a pot of water that is filled to about the same line as the contents of the mason jar, and heat until just melted.) Immediately stir in the essential oils until well blended. Pour into glass or metal storage containers and let cool before sealing, covering, or using on the skin.

## Skin Protection and Healing Remedies

As the largest organ in the body, the epidermis goes through a lot. From burns and rashes, to cracking, peeling, abrasions, and open wounds, the skin needs to be taken care of and will most certainly require some R&R if you are out in the elements or away from the comforts of home. Try out these home remedies for healing, soothing, and moisturizing the skin.

## On Sunscreen

There is no recipe in this section for homemade sunscreen, because in all truthfulness, you should buy commercially made sunscreen with proper SPF. UVA and UVB shielding compounds like zinc and titanium dioxide can protect you from sun exposure, but they are not the kind of ingredients you can just buy from your corner store and can be dangerous if handled incorrectly or inhaled. What's more, you need a professional homogenizer to properly incorporate these ingredients into any base so that the level of skin protection is even throughout the lotion.

## Lip Balm

Moisturizing the skin, particularly when you are away from the comforts of home or in remote areas, is incredibly important for preventing painful cracking, blisters, and peeling. The same goes for your lips, and it's incredibly easy to make homemade lip balm. If you don't like the taste of chamomile or peppermint, you can omit the oil completely, or you can swap it for another essential oil with a flavor or aroma you prefer, like grapefruit, lavender, or sandalwood.

### Lip Balm Recipe
*Ingredients*

1 tablespoon beeswax pellets
1 tablespoon extra-virgin olive oil
2 teaspoons coconut oil
1 teaspoon shea butter
½ teaspoon pure aloe vera
4–6 drops chamomile or peppermint oil

*Method*

Using a double boiler on low heat, heat the beeswax and olive oil until just melted. (If you do not have a double boiler, you can put them in a heat-safe container like a mason jar, place the jar in a pot of water that is filled to about the same line as the contents of the mason jar, and heat until just melted.) When the wax has melted, add the coconut oil and shea butter. Whisk gently for about 30 seconds until the ingredients are melted and incorporated. Remove from the heat and immediately stir in the aloe vera and peppermint oil until blended. Pour into glass or metal storage containers and let cool before sealing, covering, or using on the skin.

## Deodorant

A bit of a luxury, but one that certainly won't hurt if you are soaked in sweat and haven't had the opportunity to shower in a few days. Make your own deodorant at home to use regularly or bring with you on your next sweaty outdoor trek. The coconut oil and the shea butter are what give the deodorants its smooth moisturizing qualities, the baking soda acts as the main deodorizer, and the cornstarch helps keep it all together. Store it in jars or just reuse an empty deodorant container.

### Deodorant Recipe
*Ingredients*

2 tablespoons coconut oil
2 tablespoons shea butter
¼ cup baking soda
¼ cup cornstarch

*Method*

Using a double boiler on low heat, heat the coconut oil and shea butter until just melted. (If you do not have a double boiler, you can put them in a heat-safe container like a mason jar, place the jar in a pot of water that is filled to about the same line as the contents of the mason jar, and heat until just melted.) Whisk gently for about 30 seconds until the ingredients are incorporated. Remove from the heat and immediately stir in the baking soda and cornstarch until blended. Spoon into glass or metal storage containers (or empty deodorant container) and let cool before sealing, covering, or using on the skin.

## Natural Bug Repellant

DEET-based products are, without argument, bug and insect kryptonite. If you prefer to avoid the chemicals of typical insect repellent, however, you can mix together this home remedy to help ward off the pests that ail you. The vodka in this recipe acts as a preservative. If you do not have witch hazel on hand, you can just swap it out for ¼ cup vodka and forego the remaining ½ teaspoon of vodka. Store the bug repellent in a spray bottle for easy application.

### Natural Bug Repellant Recipe
*Ingredients*

1 teaspoon eucalyptus oil
1 tablespoon castor oil
¼ cup witch hazel
½ cup distilled water
½ teaspoon vodka

*Method*
Combine all of the ingredients. Store in a spray bottle.

## Fire Ant Treatment

This is a bare-bones home remedy, because in the situation in which you encounter fire ants, you will want the fastest, most effective method possible to make that fiery pain stop. With some good old bleach, water, and a bit of toothpaste, you can stop the itching and continue on your way. The amount of toothpaste you use will be based on how much surface area you're covering, so you will have to eyeball it. Start with a dime-sized amount of toothpaste and increase as needed.

### Fire Ant Treatment Recipe
*Ingredients*

1 part bleach
1 part water
1 dime-sized dollop of baking soda- and peroxide-based toothpaste (like Arm & Hammer)

*Method*

Mix equal parts regular bleach and water. Apply to the bites using a clean cloth or sterile cotton swabs. The diluted bleach will reduce the initial pain. After 10 minutes or so, apply the toothpaste to the affected areas.

## Anti-Itch Cream

No matter what you've come across, be it dry skin, nasty fire ants, athlete's foot, or a poisonous plant, you'll need a soothing cream to help reduce the itching. Scratching wounds, particularly in cases of poison ivy, can cause infection as well as spread the itch-causing oils from the plant itself, so avoid scratching at all costs. One percent hydrocortisone is the cornerstone of anti-itch creams, but this one uses ingredients you can find pretty easily if you cannot get to a pharmacy. Apply the itch cream as needed, and make sure to keep the affected areas clean.

### *Anti-Itch Cream*
*Ingredients*

2 tablespoons baking soda
½ cup distilled water
juice of ½ lemon
20 drops of chamomile essential oil

*Method*

Combine the ingredients in order, mixing well. If you prefer another aroma, swap the chamomile out for 10 drops of peppermint oil.

## Colloidal Oatmeal Bath

Oatmeal baths have long been associated with soothing chicken pox and poison ivy, and for good reason. The oats help to reduce the pH levels in your skin and lessen the associated irritation. Oatmeal baths are great for eczema, poison ivy rashes, inflamed or itchy skin, and insect bites. "Colloidal" just means that the oats have been pulverized so that you are working with a fine powder rather than flaky oats. Incorporate the powder into a warm (but not hot) bath.

*Colloidal Oatmeal Recipe*
*Ingredients*

1 cup old-fashioned rolled oats (do not use instant oats)

*Method*

Pour the cup of oats into a blender or food processer. Pulse until the oats are powdery throughout, with a similar graininess to cornmeal. Fill the tub about halfway using warm water. Slowly sprinkle the oats into the bath as you fill the tub, doing so near the faucet so that the oats mix well.

# Burn Spray

When dealing with first- and second-degree burns, there are a few steps that should be taken immediately. First, get away from whatever it is that has caused the burn, be it a fire, a hot stove, a lighter, or the blazing sun. Run the burn under cool water for 30 seconds to prevent the burn from continuing to do damage (in the same way that a steak pulled from the oven still cooks for a few minutes from the heat it has absorbed, so too does your skin when it has been burned). Next, you will need to disinfect the burn, which can be done with soap and water, or this cooling spray:

*Burn Spray Recipe*
*Ingredients*

1 cup apple cider vinegar
1 cup water

*Method*

Pour ingredients into a spray bottle and shake gently. Spray on affected area, or soak a cloth with the burn spray and use as a compress over the burn.

# Aloe-Coconut Burn Salve

This cooling salve has the soothing effects of bit of aloe vera with the moisturizing qualities of coconut oil. Honey is often used as a natural disinfectant to burns because it pulls the bacteria away from the wound, so it plays a key role in this calming salve.

### Aloe-Coconut Burn Salve Recipe
#### Ingredients

¼ cup raw (unpasteurized) honey
¼ cup coconut oil
1 teaspoon beeswax pellets
½ teaspoon aloe vera gel

#### Method

Using a double boiler on low heat, heat the beeswax until just melted. (If you do not have a double boiler, you can put it in a heat-safe container like a mason jar, place the jar in a pot of water that is filled to about the same line as the contents of the mason jar, and heat until just melted.) When the wax has melted, add and melt the coconut oil, and then stir in the honey. Whisk gently for about 30 seconds until the ingredients are incorporated. Remove from the heat and immediately stir in the aloe vera gel until blended. Pour into glass or metal storage containers and let cool before sealing, covering, or using on the skin.

# II.

# FIRST AID FOR WHEN HELP ISN'T COMING

# CHAPTER 4

## WHEN FAUNA IS NOT YOUR FRIEND

### HOW TO TREAT AND AVOID ANIMAL ATTACKS, INSECT BITES, AND AQUATIC THREATS

ANAPHYLACTIC SHOCK

Anaphylactic shock is a serious, and often life-threatening consequence of exposure to allergens. Where *prophylaxis* refers to preventative protection, think of *anaphylaxis* as the lack thereof. While many mild irritations caused by allergens—like uncomfortable skin rashes or cold-like symptoms from exposure to pet dander—can be alleviated with antihistamines like Benadryl, antihistamines are not powerful enough to stop the aggressive, life-threatening symptoms of anaphylactic shock. The best way to cope with anaphylactic shock is to be prepared before it happens. When hospitals and medical professionals are not available or are hours away, prevention is your best antidote.

Know how to recognize the signs and symptoms of anaphylaxis, and be at the ready to act when it occurs. When life happens (as it does) and you can't prevent anaphylactic shock, arm yourself with doctor-prescribed epinephrine—the only recognized medicinal option for immediate care for anaphylaxis outside of hospitalization. Confirm your allergies and those of your family members by visiting a general practitioner and getting allergy tests. In the event you or your loved ones have severe allergies that could be potentially hazardous, your doctor will prescribe epinephrine to self-administer in these emergencies while you await medical attention.

### What Causes Anaphylactic Shock?

Anaphylaxis can be caused by a number of environmental and synthetic factors. Our bodies respond to irritants or allergens by attacking the invading substance, whether it's food or medication, and this reveals itself through a variety of uncomfortable symptoms. The immune system releases the antibody immunoglobulin (IgE), which adheres to cells and releases substances like histamines that cause intense reactions. Histamines are what we think of when we have mild allergic reactions and skin irritations, and the simple way to treat them is by taking *anti*histamines (like Benadryl). While that is pretty straightforward, histamines are not the only substances released during anaphylactic shock, so the process of treating it is not so simple as popping a Benadryl.

The most common allergic reactions or hypersensitivities causing anaphylaxis are from insect stings or bites, including those of bees, wasps, hornets, yellow jackets, and spiders; foods like shellfish, tree nuts, sesame seeds, fruit, and legumes (peanuts); medications like aspirin; non-steroidal inflammatory drugs (NSAIDs) like ibuprofen; antibiotics such as penicillin; iodine-containing dyes used when getting an X-ray; anesthetics, opioids, blood transfusions, latex, and even intense exercise following direct exposure to allergens. While these pretty intense, potentially fatal reactions can be rare and are easily avoidable for those who do not have severe allergies (e.g., only about one in 1,000 people are actually allergic to honeybees), you should never assume that you are immune to the causes of anaphylaxis simply because you have never been a victim of it or are unaware of your allergy status. An anaphylactic event *must always* be taken seriously and treated immediately.

## What Are the Signs and Symptoms of Anaphylactic Shock?

While the movie industry has informed us that severe allergic reactions occur in the form of throat closure and puffy eyes, there are myriad additional manifestations of anaphylactic shock that can be harder to recognize if you are not paying attention or are unaware of what they look like. Reactions can develop seconds after contact with an allergen, but sometimes symptoms can take anywhere from two to twelve hours to rear their heads. Many times anaphylaxis has what is called a protracted reaction, meaning that symptoms persist even with medical attention. Other times it will be a biphasic reaction, meaning that symptoms can arise and then disappear entirely, only to return in the following eight to seventy-two hours. Victims of anaphylactic shock should always be monitored well after their symptoms have subsided—at least twenty-four hours—to be safe.

### Mouth

The victim may experience tingling, itching, swelling, or a combination of these symptoms in the lips or tongue. These reactions can inflame heavily enough to block airways, so it is important to attack these symptoms head on and to do so very quickly.

### Throat and Respiration

The most severe reactions are the ones that affect breathing pathways. They can be potentially fatal if not treated right away. Coughing, wheezing, itching, shortness of breath, hoarseness, tightness of the throat, and throat closure are all severe anaphylactic reactions that require immediate attention.

### Skin Irritation

Itching, redness, puffiness, swelling, hives, and angioedema (swelling present under the skin) are all telltale signs of anaphylaxis.

### Heart

Rapid heartbeat and weak pulse are both symptoms of anaphylaxis, usually paired with other aggressive symptoms.

### Digestion

Diarrhea, cramping, nausea, and vomiting can be contributing symptoms of anaphylaxis.

### Head

Dizziness, confusion, anxiety or panic, and fainting or unconsciousness are all signs that can be related to anaphylactic shock. Some of these are self-perpetuating—allowing yourself to panic will only make matters worse, so it is important to remain calm and try to keep even breathing while assessing your situation. Keep in mind that fainting can occur for reasons other than an allergic reaction. A person who has fainted and who is not experiencing anaphylaxis is more likely to have very low heart rate, extremely pale appearance, and no respiration problems, whereas someone experiencing an allergic reaction will be flushed and have other symptoms, like skin irritation and trouble breathing.

## Treating Anaphylactic Shock

When anaphylactic shock occurs, you should address the problem immediately. Whether you or someone else is the victim, take care to remain calm, keep even breathing, and assess your situation. The only antidote to anaphylaxis is epinephrine (the hormone adrenaline), most widely known by the brand name EpiPen. In the United States, a doctor must prescribe epinephrine, but Canada supplies it over the counter. Depending on your health insurance status, epinephrine can range from manageable to prohibitive in price, but many websites offer coupons. The manufacturer of EpiPen (Mylan) offers a program that reduces co-pays to as little as zero dollars. You can also find regular vials of generic epinephrine, but this will require a syringe and should only be used with proper training. Always have a backup dose of epinephrine.

Epinephrine is your first line of defense, but it should not be the only one: if you have access to medical care, don't mess around. Seek out a hospital or medical professional if they are available to you. If these resources are no longer available, follow the instructions for use of the EpiPen, monitor the symptoms for at least twenty-four hours, and have an extra EpiPen in case of a second wave of symptoms.

### Epinephrine Dosing

A typical dose of epinephrine is 0.3mg for adults and 0.15mg for children weighing less than sixty-six pounds. Auto-injector devices like EpiPens are the best ways to administer epinephrine. EpiPens come in two different colors to help distinguish between adult dosage and children's, and are designed so that you cannot see the needle (for those who are squeamish). EpiPens have an official shelf life of a year, and are always packaged with two doses in the event of persisting or returning reactions, as well as a "trainer" without medicine to practice using the device. You can order a trainer for free on Mylan's website.

### Administering an EpiPen

Read the instructions for your device before use, and familiarize yourself with any warnings or side effects. To administer an EpiPen or similar device, inject it into the muscle of your *outer* upper thigh. DO NOT inject it into your veins, finger, toes, hands, feet, or buttocks. A medical professional should only administer additional doses beyond the first two

EpiPen devices. If vital signs are stable and symptoms of anaphylactic shock have subsided after twenty-four hours, you or the victim should be in the clear, but it is important to remain alert in the event that this changes.

## SNAKE AND LIZARD BITES

As with most dangerous creatures, you are far less likely to run into trouble if you do not go looking for it. When it comes to hazardous snakes and lizards, it's important to know what you are up against and what to do in the event of a bite. While North Americans are far less likely to run into boa constrictors or anacondas (unless you hit the everglades or know any exotic snake enthusiasts), there are several varieties of smaller but still very deadly snakes. In North America, the most common venomous snakes are **coral snakes, pit vipers,** and **copperheads.** Poisonous lizards native to North America are the **Gila monster** and the **Mexican beaded lizard**. If you live in Maine, Alaska, or Hawaii, congratulations! These are the only states that do not have poisonous snakes living naturally in the wild.

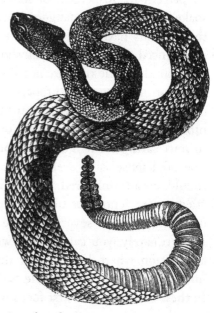

Incidents of snakebites tend to creep up in the warmer months, and snakes are more often active at night. They prefer to hide in wooded areas, abandoned shelters, hollow logs, under rock piles, in caves, and other areas where they are protected. Like most situations, it is always wise to be careful of your footing and where you put your hands if you are walking, climbing, digging, or moving brush. Snakes do not have outer ears, so they are more likely to know you are near from vibrations in the ground. When walking through wooded areas, it is a good idea to walk heavily to announce your presence

*A rattlesnake.*

to any possible snakes. Wear hiking boots or other protective footwear, long pants and sleeves, and even thick gloves.

## When Snakes Attack

When in a wooded area or an area with a known snake population, be prepared. Avoid consuming alcohol or recreational drugs that may impair your ability to react or get yourself out of danger quickly. If you come across a snake, do not provoke it. Snakes are territorial and will lash out. While avoiding venomous snakes is best practice, accidents do happen. In the event of a bite, be aware that snakes are not one-and-done: they won't just let go and die or slither away after they have bitten you. Some may cling to the wound to release as much venom as possible, while others may back off quickly only to lash out again. They do not release all of their venom in one bite, so they still pose a threat even if they have already bitten you. Even snakes that have been killed or beheaded can still continue to bite reflexively for as long as ninety minutes afterward, so it is important to stay clear of dead snakes. Roughly 35 percent of venomous snakebites are mild in potency, 25 percent are moderate in potency, and 10 percent to 15 percent are reported as severe or life-threatening. About 25 percent to 30 percent of snakebites are dry bites, meaning that the snake has not released dangerous venom. If you have been bitten and eight to ten hours have passed without incident, it is likely that you simply experienced a dry bite, but you should still continue to treat and monitor the wound. While they are not always venomous, open wounds still pose a risk for infection if not properly cleaned and tended to.

If a venomous snake or lizard bites you or someone you are with, be proactive. Do not wait for signs or symptoms that the bite is dangerous to start caring for it. For venomous snakes, the first and most effective line of defense is to seek medical care and get antivenin. Antivenin should be administered within four hours of the bite, but it can be effective for venomous bites for up to two weeks after an initial attack, depending on the severity of the bite and the potency of the venom. Unfortunately, you cannot just whip up antivenin in your kitchen. In a situation where hospitals or doctors are no longer an option, it is unlikely that you will be able to find it or obtain it for long-term use. In these scenarios, the first focus will instead be on how not to make the situation worse.

## Signs and Symptoms of a Venomous Bite

- The wound burns or stings
- Fever
- Swelling, discoloration, or rash on the skin
- Pus or excessive bleeding
- Blood in the urine
- Bleeding from gums or nose
- Muscle and joint aches
- Numbness and tingling of wound, mouth, or tongue
- Metallic taste in the mouth
- Slowed speech and disorientation
- Difficulty breathing or swallowing
- Twitching
- Paralysis

### Caring for Venomous Snake and Lizard Bites

For starters, you or the victim should remain calm. If you can evacuate to find professional medical care, do so slowly and with caution to keep the heart rate down. If this is not an option, make sure you are no longer under threat of attack. Take deep, slow breaths and try to keep the heart rate normal. Stress and a rapid heart rate will only facilitate increased blood circulation, which will enable the venom to spread even faster. Lie down, and keep the attacked limb as still as possible. Most snakebites occur on the feet, ankles, hands, and arms. If the bite is on a limb, make sure that the extremity in question is positioned *lower* than the heart. This will help slow down the circulating venom. Do not use tourniquets or wrap the bite tightly in compression bandages. Remove any jewelry, such as watches, rings, hair ties, or bracelets in case of swelling in the affected area. Some swelling can spread all the way up a limb, so keep this in mind. For example, if you are bitten on the hand and are wearing a shirt with tight sleeves, remove the shirt or cut the sleeves before swelling occurs.

Do not cut the bite open. While cowboy and outdoorsman methods of yore assured us that sucking the wound clean and spitting out the venom guaranteed survival, this is actually false. Do not suck the wound or use any venom extraction tools to pull venom from the open bite—it's too late, and it will only aggravate the wound. Put pressure on it to stop the bleeding, and then clean the punctures with mild soap and water. Check the bite for teeth. Some snakes lose their fangs during the struggle of a bite, so if necessary, carefully remove these from the wound with tweezers. Draw a circle around the circumference of the wound, and do this again every fifteen minutes to monitor how rapidly the bite is swelling or spreading. If the wound worsens, you will be able to tell with each ring that you draw around it.

Make sure the bite is clean, that any dirt and debris has been removed, and then apply a bandage. If the bandage gets wet or dirty, replace it with a new one. Shallow puncture wounds tend to heal pretty quickly, so it is okay to skip the bandage for minor bites as long as the bleeding has stopped and you keep the wound clean and out of harm's way. Set the limb in a firm splint to help prevent unnecessary movements. Use bandages or any available clothing to tie the ends of the splint so that it stays in place. When securing the splint, make sure to wrap the ends of the splint tightly, but not too tightly that you cut off circulation. Continue to monitor the wound and any alarming symptoms that may arise from the attack for several days, if not a couple of weeks.

## Snake and Lizard Bite DOs

- DO get away from the venomous snake or lizard
- DO seek medical help for antivenin
- DO remain calm
- DO lie still
- DO restrict movement to the limb
- DO remove jewelry or any tight clothing
- DO clean the wound with soap and water
- DO ice the wound, but not directly on the skin
- DO take the recommended dose of acetaminophen (Tylenol) for pain relief if necessary
- DO monitor all severe symptoms intently for the next few days, but remain vigilant for up to two weeks

## Snake and Lizard Bite DON'Ts

- DON'T suck the venom from the wound or use an extractor
- DON'T do anything to increase your blood pressure
- DON'T wrap a compression bandage or tourniquet around the wound
- DON'T apply iodine, rubbing alcohol, or hydrogen peroxide to the wound
- DON'T take blood-thinning pain relievers like aspirin or ibuprofen (NSAIDs), as this will prevent blood from clotting and delay healing
- DON'T soak the wound in ice and risk tissue damage

## Common North American Poisonous Snakes and Lizards

### Coral Snakes

Often mistaken for the king snake, the coral snake is brightly colored with black, yellow, and red bands of scales and has a black snout. The old adage goes, "Red touch yellow, kill a fellow / Red touch black, friend of Jack" (or "venom it lacks"). This is only handy in some cases of North American coral snakes, as it is not a hard and fast rule, so always proceed with caution. The symptoms of coral snakebites are neurotoxic, meaning that you or the victim will experience problems like slowed or slurred speech, disorientation, nerve damage, and paralysis from the potent venom if not treated immediately.

### Pit Vipers

There are hundreds of subspecies of pit vipers, but the most commonly known ones in North America are **rattlesnakes, cottonmouths** or **water moccasins,** and **copperheads.** They are given the name pit viper because of the presence of a heat-sensing pit organ. Located between the eyes and nostrils, this receptor helps the snake size up potential prey. Generally, pit vipers have catlike eyes and triangular heads. Within an hour of a pit viper bite, symptoms can include blistering, bruising, bleeding from gums and nose, fever, chills, and blurred vision.

- **Rattlesnake**
  - o recognized by their rattles and earth-tone skin
- **Cottonmouth** or **Water Moccasin**
  - o semi-aquatic and found in the southeastern United States
  - o brown, black, or gray in color; hourglass patterns on the skin
- **Copperheads**
  - o range in color, but mostly earth tones like brown, tan, pink, and copper; skin has lateral bands
  - o freeze when confronted by a predator (you), then attack
  - o bite repeatedly

## *Gila Monster*

The Gila monster (pronounced *hee-lah*), is a carnivorous reptile found in desert regions of the southwestern United States and northern Mexico. They are one of the largest lizards in North America, ranging from one to two feet long, with stumpy legs, a thick tail, and easily recognizable abstractly patterned skin. They are usually black with yellow, orange, or pink features. It is one of the few lizards in the world that is venomous, and while its venom is on the lesser end of the potency scale, its bites can be extremely vicious. Snakes inject venom into their victims with their fangs, but Gila monsters bite the victim and hold on as they chew. Their venom gets released from salivary glands during this process, which runs down grooves in their teeth and into the wound. It can be extremely difficult to remove the lizard once attached, and struggling can cause more tissue damage. Gilas will not typically attack unless they are being held or taunted, so the best prevention is to stay away before you can provoke them.

## *Mexican Beaded Lizard*

Much like its Gila monster relative, the Mexican beaded lizard is a large, short, and powerful venomous lizard. It can be found in Mexico and parts of southern Guatemala. Its skin is less vibrant in color than the Gila, with black beaded scales that have yellow or gray details. It is generally between two and three feet long, making it significantly larger than the Gila monster. The Mexican beaded lizard passes venom in a similar way as the Gila monster, by biting the victim and releasing the venom over the grooves of its teeth rather than by injecting it from fangs. Both the Gila monster and the Mexican beaded lizard feed on eggs and spend much of their time underground, so running into one is less likely, but not unheard of. Do not provoke this lizard, as a bite is extremely painful—it will hold on as it bites and can tear at the skin and muscle tissue, which is only further aggravated by its burning venom.

## INSECT BITES

## Bee Stings

The hazards of bee stings range from mild and manageable to life-threatening. In situations when you or a family member have been stung just once or a few times and there is no worry of an allergic reaction, it is actually quite easy to treat the sting. Encountering bee hives, colonies, or swarms is a different story. You will need to know how to prepare for such events, have an exit strategy, and seek medical attention.

### *The Deal with Bees*

Bees are like landlords: they hate loud noises, commotion, potent smells, and will waste no time protecting their property. When near a hive or out in the woods where you are unsure of the location of hives, it's important to respect the land around you. Avoid wearing heavy colognes or perfumes, stay on a path or in clear areas where you can see your footing, and do not swat at bees or attempt to destroy hives. All of these things have the potential to provoke an attack. Wear bright or lighter colors; bees tend to associate darker colors (such as red, black, and brown) and certain textures (like fur or leather) as predatory—they will assume you are a bear or other potential threat to their hive.

Bees build their nests in all kinds of locations, from gutters and the undersides of porches, to trees and holes near water sources and the undersides of rocks. This means that you are better served not putting your hands where your eyes can't see—you never know if a colony lies in wait. Bees become more aggressive the older they are and the larger their colony is. Africanized honey bees (a.k.a. "killer bees") are particularly vicious. Bees will not bother you if you don't bother them, but if they feel threatened, they will attack. While the bee that stings you *will* die, bees can smell their dead and this essentially acts as a call for backup.

### *Localized Bee Sting*

In the event of a localized bee sting, when you only have to treat one or two stings and there is no longer a threat, treatment is relatively simple. The sting will cause mild (but lingering) pain, swelling, and redness, and there will be a wheel surrounding the wound. Swelling is normal, even if the swelling surrounds the larger area around the sting. However, swelling that expands to other parts of your body is a sign of a more serious allergic reaction.

## Attack by Swarm

Whether you are severely allergic to bees or not, being attacked by a swarm of honeybees, wasps, or the like can be life-threatening. It's important to know how to get away and stay away from groups of bees in order to avoid being stung or overwhelmed by the swarm. While this doesn't mean you should be overconfident when encountering an active hive, people have a surprising ability to endure bee stings. Most people can suffer ten stings per pound of body weight and still be okay. This means that adults can be attacked and suffer more than one thousand stings without dying, and children can handle about five hundred. Being attacked a thousand times may be possible, but obviously, it's probably the last thing you want to do.

If you are attacked by a swarm of bees, the most important thing to do is run. Put as much distance between yourself and the hive or group of bees as you possibly can until you find shelter. Cover sensitive areas like your face, eyes, and throat with clothing. Pull your shirt over your head as you run if you have to. If you can't get away, cover yourself completely with clothing or blankets to protect from stinging. Erratic movement aggravates bees, so try not to swat or flail as you run. If you are near a body of water: do not under any circumstances jump into that water. Bees will hover over the surface until you come back up, and even if you have the lung capacity of a Navy SEAL, the threat will still be there when you finally resurface.

## Bee Swarm DOs

- RUN
- Protect and cover your face and head
- Do not swat or flail
- Keep running until you find shelter
- If you cannot find shelter, cover whole body with blankets
- Do not jump in water to hide from bees
- In the event of anaphylaxis, use a doctor prescribed EpiPen

### Treating Bee Stings

The first course of action is to remove the stinger and to clean the wound with soap and water. The sooner you remove the stinger, the better, because this will prevent more venom from getting into your skin that will just cause more pain. While you can remove the stinger with tweezers, the stingers still have venom in them, so tweezing can actually squeeze more venom into your wound. Instead, scrape the stinger off your skin with a flat-edged instrument, such as your fingernail, a credit card, or a dull knife.

Use ice or a cold pack wrapped in a towel to ice the wound for ten minutes at a time to reduce pain and swelling. Be careful not to freeze your skin. Drink water to hydrate, and take an antihistamine like Benadryl or Claritin to reduce swelling, redness, and itching. If the pain is too much or persists, take a recommended dose of ibuprofen (Advil or Motrin) or acetaminophen (Tylenol). Calamine lotion or 1 percent hydrocortisone cream will also help deal with swelling, itching, and pain associated with the sting. Other remedies to alleviate pain and clean the wound include rubbing the area with small amounts of vinegar, tea tree oil, baking soda paste, honey, or toothpaste (although not all combined).

If a swarm attacks you or your companion, or if there is an allergy, medical attention will be absolutely necessary. If you can get to a hospital or find a doctor, do this. If not, then you will need to treat for anaphylactic shock and administer epinephrine; disinfect, ice, and soothe the stings, and do everything possible to stay calm and try to keep yourself or your companion comfortable. (See section on anaphylactic shock beginning on page 61.)

## Black Widow Spiders

The black widow spider carries an ominous reputation for a reason. Found primarily in the western United States and parts of western Canada (often rural and suburban areas), the black widow can survive in both extremely hot desert conditions and high-altitude mountainous regions. Black widows are reclusive, meaning that they tend to bite defensively when their webs have been disturbed. Pair this with the fact that black widows like to nest in low-to-the-ground spaces like garages, holes, rock walls, or near swimming pools, and it is likely that you have or will stumble across one or many in this part of the country.

Female black widows tend to bite with more venom than males, and can be identified easily: their shiny black bodies are about half-an-inch long, or about one and a half inches including their long legs. Black widows are identifiable by an hourglass shape on the underside of their bellies that can be red, orange, or yellow. While the hourglass is the telltale mark of a black widow, it can also just appear as one large dot or two smaller dots that are not connected. Male black widows look almost nothing like the females, other than their long and sharp-looking legs. They are usually tan or brown with occasional darker or lighter flecks of the same color.

The bite of a black widow is not particularly vicious—it may just feel like a sharp pinprick. While bites from the males should certainly be taken seriously, it is the female bite that carries more venom and is more medically hazardous. The affected area will appear red or streaky after the initial bite (though it is unlikely to swell), sometimes exhibiting two small fang marks. Symptoms will usually appear within an hour, which can include local pain, sweating, headache, high blood pressure, flu-like symptoms such as chills and fever, shock, and, notably, muscle cramps near the bite and abdominal pain or rigidity. As a neurotoxin, black widow venom can cause even more severe reactions, like localized paralysis and numbness. Black widow bites are treatable, but it is important to remain calm and limit activity that will increase blood flow and therefore help circulate the venom. Children are much more likely to suffer more severe—or life-threatening—symptoms from black widow bites. Black widow bites can be severe, but they are not necessarily a death sentence; they often come with mild flu-like symptoms that can be treated at home. However, they should still be taken seriously and you should always seek medical attention if it is available to you. Ice the bite and seek antivenin, which is widely available for black widow bites.

The best way to prevent black widow bites is to reduce clutter in your home, regularly vacuum to prevent cobwebs and spider webs from forming, seal up cracks in the foundation, and keep woodpiles away from the house. Always wear gloves when moving wood to and from woodpiles, as this is a regular hangout for black widows. Regularly keep storage bins tightly sealed and clutter-free in garages or sheds, clean off the spider webs from outdoor furniture, and be vigilant about cleaning off plastic children's toys with crevices or hollow spaces (like toy cars, swing sets, and toy kitchen units). Spraying repellent and pesticides is not the most effective preventative measure with spiders unless the spider or its web is sprayed directly. Even then, it may take several hours or days for the spider to succumb to the pesticide. If you find a black widow spider in your home, you can remove it by vacuuming the web and the spider with it, crushing it (do not do this barefooted), or covering it with a jar and sliding it onto a piece of paper so you can release it at least one hundred feet away from your home.

## Ticks

These parasites are nuisances whether you are trying to prevent tick bites, remove a tick that has already bitten an individual, or deal with the medical consequences of a tick bite that has led to Lyme disease, Colorado tick fever, or malaria-like babesiosis. Both hard ticks (*Ixodidae*) and soft ticks (*Argasidae*) require blood to survive, and do so by latching on to a victim's skin and consuming blood over the course of several hours. Ticks, prior to feeding, can be as small as a seed and are usually tan or brown in color. Adult ticks have eight legs, and their mouths have several different parts that all work together to keep the tick latched on during feeding. Ticks have two chelicerae, which serve to cut through the skin, and one hypostome, which is like a barbed needle through which they eat. The barbs on this mouthpiece have the same effect on human skin as a fishhook so that it is very difficult to remove or interrupt the feeding process. Since they cling when they bite, removing them is particularly difficult and can do more harm than good if the removal is done sloppily.

### Lyme Disease

While tick bites can be harmless, they can sometimes lead to the transfer of Lyme disease in the bitten individual. If hard ticks are removed within twenty-four to thirty-six hours of the bite, it is unlikely that the victim will become infected with Lyme disease. Soft ticks generally only stay latched on for about thirty minutes, and can cause recurring fever in the individual if they have transmitted disease. A normal sign of a tick bite—though not an indicator of Lyme disease—is a red bump where the tick bit the skin. In the case of Lyme disease, a rash will begin to form any time from three to thirty days after the initial bite. The rash will expand outward and clear up in the center, forming what is often referred to as a bull's-eye pattern. The rash can grow as large as a foot in diameter. While the rash will not be itchy or feel irritated, the victim may experience flu-like symptoms such as head and body aches, fever, chills, and fatigue. Lyme disease can result in serious health problems if left undiagnosed and untreated. Long-term symptoms can be manifested as joint pain or inflammation, spread of the rash, and even neurological problems like numbness, paralysis, facial palsy, or meningitis. Rarely, infected individuals can experience fatigue, eye inflammation, and irregular heartbeat.

## Removing and Treating Tick Bites

Ticks are most often found in wooded and grassy areas. When you are in a forested, grassy, or other area where you expect to come into contact with a lot of brush, you should be careful to cover your skin entirely and check for ticks often. Wear a hat, gloves, long sleeves, and tuck your pants bottoms into your socks whenever possible while in areas that could have a higher concentration of ticks. Protect yourself with insect repellents that contain DEET, which can greatly reduce the incidence of tick bites. When leaving an area that may have ticks, make sure to check your legs, arms, scalp, groin, underarms, and any other part of the body that may have come into contact with ticks. Inspect pets as well, as they may have ticks clinging to their coats and create the possibility of transfer to humans.

Removing ticks from the skin is a careful process and should not be done hastily. With a commercially sold tick remover or a pair of fine-point tweezers, clamp onto the mouth area of the tick. This will probably include a bit of skin to ensure that complete extraction occurs. Pull the tick straight outward so that the tick's body does not rip away from the parts holding onto the skin. Do not squeeze the body of the tick, as this can cause infectious fluids to spurt back into the victim. Burning the tick or applying petroleum jelly, glue, and nail polish are all ineffective ways to remove ticks, because you need to completely extract the barbed mouthparts. Ice the bite to help ease any local discomfort. Heat kills ticks, so it is good practice to put clothes that have or may have ticks on them in the dryer for at least fifteen minutes.

If the tick is no longer attached to the skin but there is a red bump or you suspect you have been bitten, you will want to monitor the potential bite closely and seek medical attention. At the first site of the bite, draw a circle around the outer edges with a permanent marker. If the redness spreads beyond the circumference of the circle you have drawn in the coming hours or days, it is very likely that you or the individual in question has contracted Lyme disease.

In the event you think you have Lyme disease, the best thing to do is to contact a medical professional and get a diagnosis. This is usually done with the ELISA (enzyme-linked immunosorbent assay) test and the Western blot test. Early stage Lyme disease can be treated with approximately fourteen to twenty-one days of oral or intravenous antibiotics like doxycycline for adults and children over eight years old, and amoxicillin for adults, pregnant or breast-feeding women, and young children.

## Fire Ants

Fire ants are nasty, ferocious, and have the unpleasant tendency to swarm. When they bite an individual, they are capable of doing so many times, and can release venom than can cause a number of reactions, from the mild to the life-threatening. Fire ants will bite repeatedly, injecting more and more venom each time that causes a severe stinging or burning sensation. If you have disturbed a fire ant nest, you will have very little time to react. The fire ants will go on the offensive immediately, scaling any vertical surface (you) immediately in a large swarm. In this event, the first thing to do is put as much space between you and the nest and swarm of fire ants as possible. If the fire ants are climbing on you, use an article of clothing to swiftly swat them off your skin as you run away. You will want to keep doing this until you are out of danger, and you should remove your clothing to make sure there are no fire ants hiding in pockets or creases. Like ticks, it is a good idea to put your clothing in the dryer for at least fifteen minutes to kill any leftover fire ants.

Fire ant bites have a harsh burning sensation and will create swollen, itchy bumps in the affected areas within the first hour. Treat the area with a topical antihistamine to reduce discomfort, elevate the affected area, and ice the stings on and off every fifteen minutes with a towel between the ice and your skin. (Icing the skin directly can cause tissue damage.) After several hours or a day, the bites will mostly likely turn into swollen pustules filled with dead tissue. These small blisters cannot be prevented by application of topical treatment, may burst, and may leave scars. If the fluid-filled blisters burst, clean the area thoroughly with soap and water and treat with antibacterial ointment to reduce the risk of infection. Severe reactions can include anaphylaxis (including swelling of the tongue and throat), hives, nausea, diarrhea, and difficulty breathing. For severe allergic reactions and anaphylaxis, use of an EpiPen (epinephrine) may be required. If you have access to medical care, do so immediately.

## Aquatic Threats

### Stingrays

Stingray injuries are incredibly painful and in very rare circumstances can lead to death. The stingray's barbed stinger can do significant damage, as the barb itself is made up of tiny, sharp spines capable of puncturing skin and severing arteries, and it will break off and embed into a wound upon stinging. (Like a fingernail, the barb can grow back.) The stinger contains venom, which can cause swelling, intense pain, and muscle cramping in the local wound. In famous fatal cases, such as the death of Steve Irwin, it was not the stinger's venom that led to death, but rather because the stinger severed the thoracic wall. Open wounds from stingray injuries tend to bleed profusely, and it often takes a while to control and stop the bleeding. Once stung, the most severe pain will last for thirty to sixty minutes, and can continue for up to forty-eight hours. The victim may experience chills, headaches, nausea, fever, and fatigue.

Stingrays are not aggressive sea creatures and will only sting defensively. In most cases, they sting because they have been stepped on. When you are in an area that may be populated by stingrays, proceed through the water with caution and drag your feet through the sand. The disruptions in the sand will alert the stingrays of your presence and usually they will move without incident. If you or a companion has been stung, the first thing to do is to rinse the wound with the salt water, clearing away any dirt and particles from the barb (if the barb is deeply embedded, wait for professional emergency services). When the victim has been removed from the water, pour hot water (45°C/113°F) over the wound to deactivate the venom and soothe the affected area. Be careful not to burn the skin. Seek medical attention, as the wound will need to be thoroughly cleaned and assessed. Keep the wound elevated and bandage it with clean gauze.

## Jellyfish

Jellyfish are extremely powerful creatures, in the sense that their stings can be deadly and agonizingly painful, but also because even if they have washed ashore and are dying, they are still plenty capable of stinging anyone that comes into contact with them. Jellyfish stings are so harmful because the tentacles release millions of nematocysts, which penetrate the skin and inject painful venom. While most jellyfish stings are not deadly or even necessarily painful, stings from certain classes of jellyfish (e.g., box jellyfish, like the sea wasp or Irukandji) can be excruciating and cause death within minutes. Another danger is the victim going into shock while still in the water, which can cause drowning.

When stung by a jellyfish, the first thing to do is to get away from the water. Water, particularly fresh water, triggers the activity of the nematocysts, which can cause more harm by releasing additional venom. Pour vinegar of 4 percent to 6 percent acetic acid on the affected area to deactivate the nematocysts and relieve some of the stinging. When treating a jellyfish victim, wear gloves or wrap your hands in wet suit material or pantyhose to block the nematocysts. Gently scrape off the jellyfish stingers using a sharper edge, like a credit card, razor, or shell found in the sand. If you happen to have baby powder available, sprinkle it over the affected area to help facilitate the removal of the stingers. Do not use alcohol, ammonia, or urine to clean jellyfish stings. In areas where harmful jellyfish tend to reside, wear a wet suit or pantyhose while swimming to help protect you from the sting.

# CHAPTER 5

# THE ENVIRONMENT STRIKES BACK

## WHAT TO DO WHEN MOTHER NATURE GOES AGAINST YOU

### POISONOUS PLANTS

Poisonous plants fall into two categories: the kinds that cause sickness, and sometimes death, through ingestion and the kinds that can cause a severe skin reaction merely by touch. Proper plant identification and avoidance is the key to avoiding getting ill in the first place. In the case of ingesting poisonous plants, this especially means only eating plants you have identified with certainty. Common poisonous plants often mimic the look of edible plants. However, this also means sticking to the parts of a plant that are known to be safe. Apples, for example, are perfectly safe to eat, but in significant quantities their seeds, which contain cyanide, can be incredibly harmful.

In the case of plants where transference occurs by direct, physical touch rather than consumption, wearing clothing that covers most of the body and washing after spending time outside in areas that are likely to have these plants is helpful.

### Belladonna (a.k.a. Deadly Nightshade)

The dark, glossy, black single berries (as opposed to the cluster berries of raspberries) are very similar in appearance to edible elderberries, and they can also be mistaken with wild blueberries to the incautious eye. Unlike elderberries and blueberries, however, nightshade is incredibly toxic, though what constitutes a lethal dose is still uncertain. There's at least one case of a small child dying after ingesting only half a berry, while a Danish nine-year-old survived after eating between twenty to twenty-five nightshade berries mixed in with blueberries.

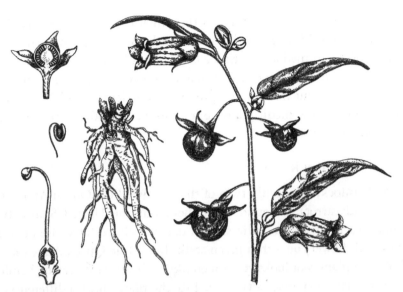

*Atropa belladonna, or deadly nightshade.*

It's also important to note that while belladonna is arguably the most toxic of the nightshades, all nightshade plants—a category that includes potatoes, eggplants, bell peppers, and tomatoes—are toxic. The fruits are safe to eat, but one should not eat the leaves, roots, or stems.

### What Makes Nightshade So Deadly?

Nightshades have potent enzyme inhibitors that interfere with the body's natural processes, including neurological ones.

### What Are Symptoms of Nightshade Poisoning?

Symptoms can be slow to appear but last for several days and include dryness, incredible thirst, difficulty swallowing and speaking, and slurred speech. The poison causes pupils to dilate, leading to blurred vision and sensitivity to light. Additionally, those suffering from nightshade poisoning will experience vomiting, a racing heartbeat, slurred speech, confusion, disorientation, and delirium. Convulsions and a coma typically precede death.

### How Do You Treat Nightshade Poisoning?

The traditional medical treatment for nightshade poisoning is physostigmine (itself somewhat lethal), which occurs naturally in the Calabar bean, and pilocarpine, a parasympathomimetic alkaloid obtained from the leaves of the *Pilocarpus* or jaborandi bush. Absent access to these, the patient should immediately drink a large glass of warm vinegar or a mixture of mustard and water, which may dilute and neutralize its toxicity. After that, it's about treating symptoms. The patient should drink plenty of fluids and follow medical advice for specific symptoms. Seek medical attention when possible.

## Poison Hemlock

Poison hemlock, the deadly twin of the wholly edible Queen Anne's lace (a.k.a. wild carrot), is found throughout out the United States. Both plants present as an umbrella-shaped delicate cluster of white or sometimes pink flowers on a thin green stalk. But while Queen Anne's lace is edible (the plant root looks very much like a white carrot), eating hemlock is a distinctly risky proposition. Luckily the plants have a differentiator: Queen Anne's lace flowers rest upon a hairy green stem, and the flowers smell like carrots. Hemlock, in contrast, rests upon a smooth stem that's mostly green with intermittent purple splotches. The flowers smell unpleasant, especially when crushed between fingers to release the scent (wash hands afterwards).

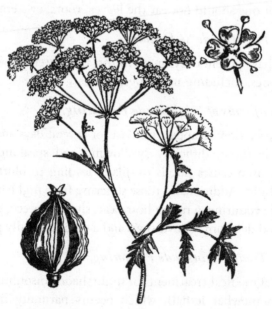

*Conium maculatum, or poison hemlock.*

### What Makes Poison Hemlock So Poisonous?

Hemlock contains a variety of alkaloids that are harmful to humans. The most critical is coniine, which causes muscle paralysis and can seriously affect the heart and respiratory system. Stripped of their ability to function, the person can eventually die of lack of oxygen to the heart or brain.

### What Are Symptoms of Poison Hemlock Exposure?

Poison hemlock toxicity usually presents itself as nervous trembling, a lack of coordination, excess saliva production, dilation of the pupils, and a rapid, weak pulse. The toxins present can affect respiration and make breathing incredibly difficult. Convulsions are not uncommon, and periodically it presents with gastrointestinal irritation and bloody bowel movements.

### How Do You Treat Poison Hemlock Exposure?

Symptoms of hemlock poisoning generally appear within twenty minutes to three hours of exposure. Treatment involves activated charcoal and a saline cathartic (to purge the system); you want the person to get as much fluids in them as possible while balancing their electrolyte load. Sports beverages mixed with water, or medical beverages like Pedialyte, are beneficial. You can also make your own beverage using a mixture of salt, sugar, and water. Poison hemlock can affect a person's breathing, so make sure you support their breathing through artificial respiration if necessary and have them positioned in such a way (upright) as to make breathing easier. Symptoms should disappear within seventy-two hours.

## The Poisonwood Trio: Poison Ivy, Poison Oak, and Poison Sumac

### Poison Ivy

Poison ivy is found throughout the United States, except in Alaska, Hawaii, and in parts of the West Coast. The rash-inducing plant can grow as a vine, a small shrub close to the ground, or climbing on low plants, trees, and poles. The plant is best identified by its leaves. Each leaf has three glossy leaflets that inspired the age-old childhood chant, "leaves of three let them be," which also applies to poison oak. The poison ivy's leaves are reddish in the spring, green in the summer, and yellow, orange, or red in the fall. Depending on the season, the plant can have greenish-white flowers and whitish-yellow berries.

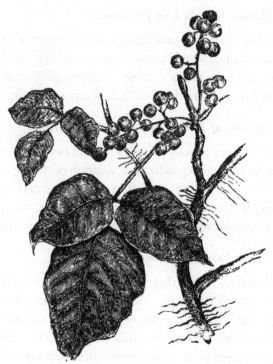

*Toxicodendron radicans, or poison ivy.*

## Poison Oak

This low shrub has fuzzy leaves that appear in clusters of three or five leaves. In the spring the leaves may be green or red, in summer the leaves are green and the plant grows deceptively pretty berries, and in fall the leaves turn red and orange. Poison oak is most prevalent in bogs or swamps in the Northeast, Midwest, and parts of the Southeast.

## Poison Sumac

Poison sumac grows as a tall shrub or small tree in wetlands across the Northeast, Midwest, and the Southeast. Its leaves appear in clusters of thirteen leaflets with smooth edges. The leaves are orange in spring, green in summer, and yellow, orange, or red in fall. The plant gets its name from the fact that it looks very similar to normal sumac, albeit with a toxic bite.

## What Makes the Poisonwood Trio So Poisonous?

The "poison" aspect of poison ivy, oak, and sumac, comes from a chemical compound called urushiol that resides on its surface. Eighty-five percent of people are allergic to it, which can lead to annoying, persistent, itchy rashes. Urushiol is also present in mango skin, though in much lower levels. Contact with the peel of mangoes can trigger a reaction in particularly susceptible individuals.

### What Are Symptoms of Poison Ivy, Oak, and Sumac Exposure?

The rash caused by poison ivy, oak, and sumac, called contact dermatitis, is the most common symptom. The rash, reddish and itchy with swelling bumps and small blisters, will form basically anywhere that has been in contact with the plant. A rash line that looks a lot like the plant line isn't uncommon. In rare cases a fever greater than 100°F can occur, and in children more severe blistering isn't uncommon. Wheezing and difficulty breathing can occur if you've breathed in burning poison ivy—after accidentally throwing it into a campfire for example. Symptoms generally appear twenty-four to forty-eight hours after exposure.

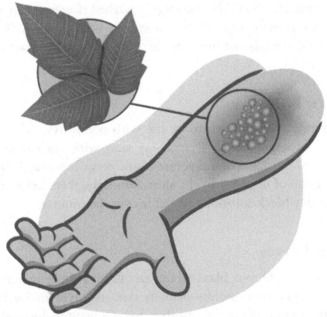

*A rash from one of the poisonwood trio.*

### How Do You Treat Poison Ivy, Oak, or Sumac Exposure?

Begin by rinsing off the exposed area with either soap and water or rubbing alcohol as quickly after exposure as possible. After fifteen minutes of contact, the oils become bonded to the skin and a reaction is all but guaranteed. After that point, soothing lotions like calamine lotion, cortisol creams, and aloe vera (fresh from the plant if you can get it), along with cool baths with colloidal oatmeal and baking soda mixed in, are the go-to treatments. Antihistamines such as oral Benadryl can help with the itching, but antihistamine creams (like Benadryl cream) can actually make things worse.

### Don't Scratch

Contrary to myth, the blisters don't spread the chemical. Scratching them, however, can cause them to become infected, which only makes things worse. Symptoms should improve within ten days.

### Wash Everything

While you can't spread the infection to yourself, clothes can harbor oils for up to a year and should be thoroughly washed after exposure to poison ivy. The same goes for any pets that may have been exposed. While they won't get sick, the oils can linger in their fur, re-exposing you every time you pet them.

### An Ounce of Prevention

If heading to an area known to be rife with poison ivy, oak, or sumac, an old forest ranger's trick is to spray skin with antiperspirant (not deodorant). Aluminum chlorohydrate in antiperspirant may help prevent the penetration of urushiol in the skin. Similarly, there are a number of pre-contact ivy block solutions available over the counter.

## Rhubarb Leaves

Rhubarb, the red fibrous plant whose tart flavor is delicious in pies and compotes, hides a toxic secret—namely that its leaves are inedible. The leaves contain a number of poisons that, in large enough dosages, can kill. This was a common problem during World War I in England, where the leaves were mistakenly recommended as a food source (other plant tops, such as beet leaves, are perfectly safe to eat).

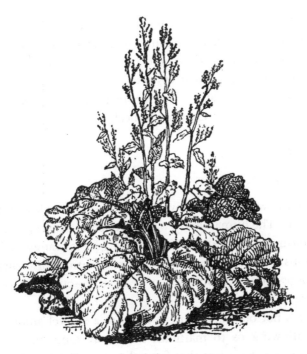

*Rheum rhabarbarum, or rhubarb plant.*

### What Makes Rhubarb Leaves So Deadly?

The leaves contain a significant amount of oxalic acid, a chemical present in many plants, including spinach, kale, and broccoli. Even the rhubarb stem that we safely eat contains oxalic acid. Rhubarb leaves, however, are a classic case of the dose makes the poison: they contain enough oxalic acid to cause kidney failure.

### What Are Symptoms of Rhubarb Leaf Poisoning?

The body might experience a general sense of weakness, as well as symptoms that traditionally come with gastrointestinal distress, including burning in the mouth and throat, nausea, stomach pain, diarrhea, and vomiting. Urine can turn red, signaling the presence of kidney stones or kidney failure. Eye pain, seizures, and coma can also follow.

### How Do You Treat Rhubarb Leaf Poisoning?

Hemodialysis is considered the baseline measure where the toxins are literally filtered out of the blood. Absent access to that level of medical care, stomach pumping (if possible—do not induce vomiting) and consumption of activated charcoal can help bind the protein. Once acute symptoms diminish, antacids should be used, and diets that are low on acid-inducing chemicals, such as gastric reflux diets that avoid acids (such as vinegar and tomatoes), hot peppers, chocolates, and fats should be followed to allow the body time to heal.

# EXTREME COLD
## Hypothermia

Hypothermia is what happens when your body loses heat faster than it can produce it. The human body was designed to function with an internal temperature of around 98.6°F, with a general range of variation of plus or minus 1°F. Some people run a little warmer or cooler, but with few exceptions—most notably when we're sick—our body works hard to keep it close to that range.

When it's hot outside, humans perform a marvel among mammals: we sweat, allowing us to maintain core body temperature even while we're moving around, a feat that few other animals can accomplish. And when it's cold outside, we shiver as a way of generating additional body heat. That said, there's a limit to how much our body can adapt; if we are too hot or cold for too long, then our body starts to shut down. We die.

When your internal temperature reaches 96°F, you have mild hypothermia. Your heart rate goes up and you start to shiver. This is your body's attempt at compensating for the weather. Your hands and feet grow numb, because they have a higher surface area to volume ratio than other parts of the body. It gets harder to perform basic tasks like fastening clothing. A sense of general fatigue and diminished cognitive abilities may follow, marking the beginning of moderate hypothermia, which means you may get frustrated with zipping up your jacket and not bother.

If you don't warm up soon, your body gives up on keeping itself warm and merely tries to survive. This stage, severe hypothermia, is where hallucinations become possible, and it's common for people to report feeling very warm despite the fact that they are indeed quite cold. Eventually, your heart rate slows to reduce the body's need for oxygen. Your breathing slows too, to one or two breaths per minute. Your skin grows pale and icy to the touch, your limbs stiffen, your pupils dilate, and you may burrow into a snow bank or whatever place you can find—a symptom known as "hide and die." You stop moving, appearing dead to the world, and if help doesn't come quickly, you will indeed die.

There is no set core temperature at which the human body automatically dies from the cold. In 1994, a two-year-old Saskatchewan girl wandered out into the cold on a night where temperatures dipped to −40°F. Despite the fact that her internal temperature dipped to 57°F, she lived (the lowest recorded core temperature in a surviving adult is 60.8°F).

The goal is to avoid taking our bodies to these extreme lows. The most common causes are either exposure to cold weather or to cold water, but the proximate cause in many causes is not dressing for the situation. Even Antarctic temperatures can be handled with appropriate clothing, and a popular tourist activity in arctic Iceland is snorkeling. Participants wear layers of thermal clothing and then a dry suit, which keeps the frigid waters away from the snorkelers' bodies.

You can maintain proper temperature through proper outfitting, which, contrary to popular belief, does not mean throwing on as many layers as possible. Too many layers when the temperature dips below freezing can be as bad as too few. When dressed too warmly, either because you're wearing too many layers or too many clothes for your heavy level of exertion, you frequently sweat. When that happens, a layer of clothing should be removed. Eventually, you'll either reduce your exertion, or the temperature will dip; either way you'll be looking to warm up even as the sweat that clings to your body is still cooling you down.

Contact your local outdoor outfitter for tips on the best ways of dressing for the different kinds of weather you plan on encountering.

### Chronic Hypothermia

Chronic hypothermia occurs when your body loses heat slowly over time due to being in accommodations that are heated below 60°F. It's especially common among the elderly, children, and other populations with impaired perceptions of the cold. Symptoms include purple or blue fingers and toes, shivering (although shivering frequently stops in chronic hypothermia), slow breathing, and confusion. Assuming that the sufferer is aware and conscious, the treatment involves slowly warming the person up by increasing the household temperature, swaddling them in warm layers of clothes and bedding, drinking warming beverages (such as tea;

avoid cold beverages), and exercise. It is preventable either through properly heating one's home or wearing suitable clothing while in the home to make up for the colder accommodations.

## Acute Hypothermia

Acute hypothermia is when a person rapidly loses body temperature either by being submerged in water (as detailed below) or by being underdressed in extremely cold situations.

## Water Submersion

Cold-water submersion often happens quickly—a crack in the ice, a slip off the shore, a trip on the deck. As quickly as it happens, it can kill. Cold water transports heat away from the body twenty-five times faster than air at the same temperature. If you fall into water that is near freezing, death can come in as little as fifteen minutes.

## Four Stages in Water Submersion

1. **Cold Shock Response (0–2 minutes)**
   Roughly lasting a minute after entering the water, cold shock refers to the effect that water has on the respiratory and cardiovascular systems. There's an automatic gasp response to the rapid skin cooling, and if the head goes under water this response can cause water to enter the lungs. Alternatively, if it's not controlled, this response can cause hyperventilation and ultimately loss of consciousness. Finally, the cold water causes the arteries to narrow (vasoconstriction). The heart has to work harder to pump the blood. In people with an underlying heart problem, this can cause cardiac arrest or a heart attack.
2. **Cold Incapacitation (2–15 minutes)**
   Vasoconstriction occurs as an attempt to preserve core temperature and protect vital organs by allowing the extremities to cool. Thus, muscle and nerve fibers won't work as well when they're cold, making it harder for you to stay afloat. Swimming becomes increasingly difficult. If you're not wearing a flotation device or if you haven't found something to help you float, you'll drown. If you are wearing a flotation device, the Heat Escape

Lessening Postures (HELP) where the arms are wrapped around the chest and the knees are tucked upward towards the chest can help. Similarly, if you're not alone, huddling together (with each group member's knees drawn to the chest) can also help.

3. **Hypothermia (15–30 minutes)**
   Depending on the water temperature, hypothermia can set in after as little as five minutes, though thirty minutes is more typical. This happens when the body's temperature reaches at or below 96°F.

4. **Circum-rescue (Peri-rescue) Collapse**
   Ranging from fainting to death, circum-rescue collapse is connected to the body's inability to maintain proper heart function, blood pressure, and core temperature due to the stress-inducing conditions of cold-water immersion or the efforts connected to the rescue itself. The key way of preventing this is to make sure that the victim remains horizontal—NOT vertical—during the rescue, or if not possible, after the rescue. Circum-rescue collapse is closely related to rewarming shock.

## Treating Mild Hypothermia

If you're wearing clothes that are wet either from submersion or from sweat, they should be removed and the skin dried. The patient should be moved to a warm, dry place (if possible) and protected from the elements if the location is not ideal. The body should be covered in blankets, hat, and heat packs to prevent more heat loss. Properly protected from heat loss, the body should recover on its own. Warming liquids can help, and the body must to be assessed for frostbite.

## Treating Moderate Hypothermia

Moderate hypothermia is treated similarly to mild hypothermia except that health-care workers may use a device to circulate warm air around the hypothermic patient's body. Similarly, the patient may be given heated IV fluids.

## Treating Severe Hypothermia

In the case of severe hypothermia, the methods used for moderate and mild hypothermia might not suffice. In addition to warming the person, health-care providers may use an IV to flush warm liquids into the person's stomach or intestines. If medical practitioners are on hand, oxygen masks and tubes can be used to provide moist, warm air, while a blood-recirculating machine may remove blood from the person's body, warm it, and reintroduce it.

## Rewarming Shock

Care needs to be taken when warming up anyone with moderate or severe hypothermia. Every year many hypothermia victims die in the process of being rescued. In 1980, sixteen Danish fishermen were rescued after being shipwrecked for ninety minutes in the frigid waters of the North Sea. All sixteen of them dropped dead when they went below the deck of the rescue ship for a hot drink. The shock of going from such a cold temperature to such a warm one killed them.

There are a few methods that can be used to prevent rewarming shock. First, the patient should be kept horizontal (prone) as much as possible, especially for patients taken from the water. Additionally, the goal is to raise the body temperature slowly: roughly 1°F every fifteen to twenty minutes.

# Frostnip

Frostnip is the first stage of frostbite. As this stage, skin turns pale or red from exposure to the cold and feels very cold to the touch. It's the first sign that your skin is too cold, and treatment is relatively straightforward: get out of the cold. As your skin warms, you may feel tingling or a bit of pain, but frostnip doesn't permanently damage the skin. In later stages of frostnip, often called superficial frostbite, the skin remains soft to the touch but it feels warm due to swelling. In this stage, treatment is similar to frostnip: get the skin out of the cold, and gently rewarm it. If the affected area is on the hands and feet, you can rewarm it by soaking in warm water (99°F–108°F, or warm to the touch of an uninjured elbow or finger). For ears, you can dip a cloth in warm water and wrap it around your ear. As the skin rewarms, you may notice that it appears blue or purple and may be accompanied by stinging, burning, and swelling. A blister filled with fluid may appear within twenty-four to thirty-six hours after rewarming the skin. Do not rewarm the area if there's a chance it will freeze again.

## Frostbite

Frostbite, unlike frostnip, can permanently damage the skin because ice crystals form within the skin, blood thickens and stops flowing, and the cells begin to die. When you have frostbite, the skin will feel waxy and firm to the touch, and you will no longer have sensation in the area. The skin will also have gray/black dead blisters. Treatment is similar to that of frostnip: soak the area in warm water (99°F–108°F), do not rewarm the area if there's a chance it will freeze again, and do not warm the area with direct heat (by placing it in front of a fireplace, or using heating pads, for example). Given that the rewarming process is frequently painful, the use of over-the-counter pain relievers like acetaminophen and ibuprofen may be helpful. Once the areas have been rewarmed, apply sterile dressing, wrapping fingers and toes individually so they don't touch. Very severe frostbite might require amputation, but it can take a few days to assess.

## Bronchospasm

Like chronic hypothermia, bronchospasms are associated with dwellings that are kept too cool, especially in dry areas. Certain individuals are more susceptible, such as those with asthma. The cold air and the lack of moisture can trigger the sudden constriction, or spasming, of the muscle in the walls of the bronchioles (passageways that carry air that passes through the nose or mouth to the lungs). The end result is that the person can struggle to breathe. Maintaining a home at an adequate temperature and using a humidifier indoors can help reduce incidences, as can using a scarf, mask, or other material place across the nose and mouth while outdoors. When you exhale, heat and moisture get trapped in the mask, so when you inhale the cold air is warmed and humidified as it travels through the mask. If symptoms don't subside when moved to a warmer, moister location, an inhaled corticosteroid is the preferred treatment.

## Immersion Foot

Immersion foot, perhaps better known as trench foot, happens when feet are kept in cold, wet socks and/or tucked into shoes or boots for days at a time. The foot emerges pale, clammy, swollen, and numb, but transforms to red and painful to the touch when warmed. Blisters can develop, creating areas for opportunistic infections. It goes without saying that prevention is the best way of dealing with trench foot. Wear properly fitting waterproof shoes, and make it a point to air out feet (and shoes) daily. If you get immersion foot, the treatment is similar to that of frostnip: rewarm feet gently in warm water (99°F–108°F). After the feet are warm, dry them thoroughly and keep dry and clean throughout the healing process. Elevating the foot has also been found to be beneficial.

## Chilblains

Chilblains, also known as pernio or perniosis, happens in some people when skin goes from cold temperature to warm temperatures quickly. Small blood vessels in the skin swell up causing itching, red patches, swelling, and blistering on extremities like toes, fingers, ears, and noses. They most commonly occur in children and the elderly in cold, humid climates. Unfortunately, chilblains respond poorly to treatment, the most common of which is a topical corticosteroid cream applied for a few days to help with swelling and itching. The area should be kept clean and bandaged to prevent secondary infections. Symptoms usually subside within three weeks. If you tend to suffer from chilblains, prevention is critical. You should make sure to keep susceptible areas, such as feet and hands, warm while exposed to the cold, and avoid foods and drugs like coffee and caffeine that can constrict blood vessels. Vasodilator medications, or drugs that keep your blood vessels opened, can be prescribed by doctors.

## How to Survive an Avalanche

On a snowy mountain or in extremely cold weather, the risk of succumbing to an avalanche is pretty unlikely. For those who do spend time in cold weather or mountainous regions, it is very important to be mindful and know best practices to help increase the chance of survival in the event of an avalanche or if snow becomes overwhelming. To begin, when traveling in areas that are prone to avalanche, have a beacon. This transmitter can signal responders to a person's location in the event of an avalanche, and improve the chance of survival exponentially.

When an avalanche is in full force, start to swim. A "swimming" motion in which one moves the arms and kick the legs can help a person stay above the snow. It is crucial to stay as close to the top of the surging snow pile as possible, because once covered, avalanche victims run the risk of disorientation, becoming immobilized in the heavy snow, and never resurfacing. Keep arms above the head; this can help first responders find people in the snow if a hand is sticking out, as well as help those stuck know which way is up.

When from the cascade has ceased, clear a pocket in front of the face for breathing and to help with orientation. In the likely event that one's hands are immobilized, spit directly into the snow. This will help clear a little room, and the direction that the spit falls due to gravity will show which way is up and down. Dig out in the opposite direction of where the spit falls.

Remain calm. Once trapped in an avalanche, there is a window of approximately fifteen minutes to carve out enough space to breathe while waiting for rescuers or attempting to dig oneself out. Struggling and panicking may cause hyperventilation and waste precious air, so keep calm and beathe evenly. If still in reach, use ski polls to chip through the snow and find open air.

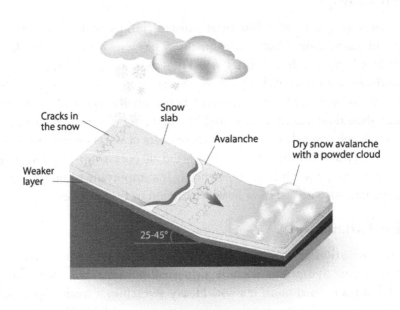

*How an avalanche forms.*

## SEVERE HEAT

Heat kills more Americans every year than any other environmental cause. While the body responds to cold by shivering (increasing the body's temperature), it deals with heat by perspiring (sweating) and breathing. Sweating works through evaporation; the water molecules use energy from your body to turn into water vapor, and this loss of energy cools the skin. But there are limits: if it's very hot or very humid (so less evaporation happens), the body can't keep up, and we overheat and die. The elderly, the very young, and people with compromised immune systems are particularly susceptible to the heat, as are people with respiratory illnesses such as asthma, because heat frequently brings with it declining air quality.

In addition, while cold can be dealt with by dressing for it, heat is best dealt with through avoidance: finding cooler shelter (such as air conditioning, shades, caves), remaining hydrated, and limiting activities (such as exercise) that will increase your body temperature when the thermometer soars above 90°F.

## Heat Cramps

Heat cramps are painful but brief muscle cramps that occur after you work or exercise in a hot environment. They can happen immediately after exertion, or a few hours later. The exact source of heat cramps is something of a mystery. They can be prevented by staying hydrated (you can tell you've drunk enough water based on the color of your urine, which should be a faint yellow) and by balancing electrolytes (the rule of thumb is one sport drink for every three units of water) while engaged in the activity and afterwards. Consumption of potassium-rich foods such as bananas and squash is also beneficial. It's important to note that heat cramps may also be a sign of heat exhaustion or heat strokes.

## Heat Exhaustion

Heat exhaustion is a heat-related illness that occurs when your body gets too hot. Symptoms include skin that is moist but cool; you get goosebumps even though it's hot. Heavy sweating, a weak, rapid pulse, exhaustion, dizziness, muscle cramps, nausea, and headache are additional symptoms. Luckily, the treatment is fairly straightforward. Stop any vigorous exercise and rest, drink plenty of fluids (both water and sports drinks or other fluids that contain salts and electrolytes), and move to a cool place. Monitor body temperature to make sure that it remains below 103°F.

## Heat Stroke

Heat stroke is the most severe of the three common heat-related ill-nesses, and potentially deadly. Heat stroke happens when the body has lost its ability to cool itself. Body temperatures reach 104°F or higher. Frequently, unless exercising, the body stops sweating and the skin is hot and dry to the touch. Other symptoms include feeling nauseous, con-fused, or disoriented. Seizures and coma are not uncommon with heat stroke, and the heart may race and breathing can become shallow and rapid. The best course of treatment is to seek medical help, but if that is out of reach, the goal is to cool the patient down quickly. Put them in a cool tub of water, or place ice packs or cold, wet towels on the person's head, neck, armpits, and groin, place them in front of a fan while you mist them with cool water.

## Prickly Heat Rash

Prickly heat rashes happen when you sweat more than normal and your sweat glands become blocked, creating a rash formed of small raised red spots with a tingling or prickly sensation (hence the name). It usually affects regions of the body that are covered by clothes, or areas of the body that rub together. Often prickly heat rash will go away on its own after a few days if the area is kept cool and dry. Avoid exercise and things that will make you sweat, refrain from scratching (colloidal oatmeal baths can help with that), and use baby powder or other drying agent in areas of the body that are prone to rub together. If it doesn't go away, over-the-counter hydrocortisone and a variety of heat rash sprays (usually contain-ing ingredients like witch hazel, lavender, and eucalyptus) can help.

## LIGHTNING

Lightning strikes happen when there's an electrical discharge from the atmosphere to the earth. They kill about twenty-four thousand peo-ple worldwide a year, but another two hundred forty thousand people are struck by lightning and survive, which is not to say that they emerge unscathed. Lightning strikes carry thousands of volts of electricity per square foot, causing severe nerve damage among survivors, many of whom report resulting memory loss, personality changes, and an inabil-ity to concentrate.

Avoidance is key to surviving a lightning strike. The Federal Emergency Management Agency (FEMA) recommends that people follow the 30/30 rule: Go indoors if, after seeing lightning, you cannot count to thirty before hearing thunder. Stay indoors for thirty minutes after hearing the last clap of thunder. 'Indoors' is not any old structure, but preferably a substantial building with wiring and plumbing that can direct charge away from occupants. Sheds, dugouts, and bus shelters actually don't offer much in the way of protection and may in fact be targets; it is better to be in a car or truck (provided that it's not a convertible) with the windows rolled up and the occupants not touching any metal parts.

If you're caught outdoors, your action depends on the location. If you're in a forest, you should seek shelter in a low area under a thick growth of small trees. Higher objects are bigger targets. If you're in an open area, you should go to a low area like a ravine or a valley while being alert for flash flooding. If you're on open water, get to land and find shelter immediately. FEMA recommends that if you feel your hair stand on end while outside, squat low to the ground on the balls of your feet, place your hands over your ears, and put your head between your knees. The goal is to make yourself into as small a structure as possible while minimizing your contact with the ground.

What if the worst happens and you do get struck by lightning? Apply standard first aid immediately. Lightning strike victims don't carry an electric charge and can't hurt anyone.

## ALTITUDE

When you move from sea level to higher altitudes, as when mountain climbing or skiing, the air becomes thinner and less oxygen is available. This is because there is less atmospheric pressure. Because lungs are effectively balloons, in order for them to inflate the air pressure in your lungs has to be less than the air pressure outside of them; the reduced pressure in high altitude environments weakens this tension making it harder to breathe. Combined, the reduction in oxygen availability and the lessened ability to breathe in as much of the oxygen that is available can lead to health complications, especially if we move from areas of low pressure to areas of high pressure too quickly.

## Altitude Sickness (a.k.a. Acute Mountain Sickness)

Altitude sickness occurs when you climb to a high altitude (generally considered anything higher than eight thousand feet above sea level) too quickly. It's most common among skiers and mountaineers, though it's becoming more common among people flying directly from places of low elevation to high elevation destinations (about twelve thousand feet).

Generally, most cases of altitude sickness are mild with symptoms such as headache, nausea, dizziness, and exhaustion. In mild cases, acclimatization will usually cause symptoms to subside. Acclimatization involves remaining at an elevation and not ascending any higher for at least forty-eight hours. If symptoms worsen or don't improve after twenty-four to forty-eight hours, you should descend by at least sixteen hundred feet.

Altitude sickness can be avoided by heading first to lower, high-altitude destinations such as those in the five to six thousand foot range (like Denver) and giving the body three to five days to adapt. In addition, you should avoid alcohol hours and exercise for the first forty-eight hours while your body adjusts.

Once above ten thousand feet, you shouldn't increase the altitude at which you sleep by more than one thousand feet a night. You can go higher during the day but it's important to go back down to a lower elevation camp at night. For example, if you're acclimatized to a location at twelve thousand feet, you could climb up to fourteen thousand feet during the day, provided you spend the night at thirteen thousand (a thousand feet above your initial elevation). Ignoring these rules can lead to high altitude pulmonary edema (HAPE) or high altitude cerebral edema (HACE), both discussed below.

It's not completely clear who is at risk for acute mountain sickness, though chest infections and any other infections that compromise one's ability to breathe will increase your risk. Apart from that, general health factors, such as degree of fitness, do not play a role. Acetazolamide, a generic prescription drug, can help speed acclimation and reduce the symptoms of acute mountain sickness while serving as additional protection if your past experiences have suggested that you might be susceptible. It can make you more sensitive to the sun, however, so it needs to be used with sunblock, and dizziness and drowsiness are known side effects. Similarly, over-the-counter medications like ibuprofen can help with headache.

Nothing is as effective, however, as simply taking your time to ascend and staying hydrated.

## High Altitude Pulmonary Edema (HAPE)

High altitude pulmonary edema (HAPE) is a severe form of mountain sickness that happens when excess fluid collects in the lung. Symptoms include a constant sense of breathlessness, even while resting, a bubbling in the chest, worsening breathlessness, and coughing up pink frothy liquid (often blood from the lungs). The best and most critical thing you can do if you think you have HAPE is to descend quickly, as much as three thousand feet. If oxygen is available, it should be given.

The standard drug treatments for which there are strong clinical evidence is the steroid dexamethasone and the calcium channel blocker nifedipine. Both require a prescription. In addition, sildenafil, better known as Viagra, and tadalafil, better known as Cialis, also work but they may make the headache associated with mountain sickness worse.

## High Altitude Cerebral Edema (HACE)

Whereas HAPE results in fluid in the lungs, high altitude cerebral edema (HACE) results in fluid in the brain. The body's normal response to a decrease in oxygen, as at high elevations, is to increase the blood flow. If blood vessels in the brain are damaged, fluid can leak out, causing HACE. Like HAPE and acute mountain sickness, it is unclear who is susceptible to HACE, though it's known that roughly 1 percent of people who ascend to elevations above ten thousand feet will develop it. It is possible to develop both HACE and HAPE simultaneously. HACE symptoms include clumsiness, difficulty walking, confusion, excessive emotion (including violence), drowsiness leading to a loss of consciousness, and, if untreated, death. Like HAPE, the best cure is descent of at least three thousand feet. The prescription drug dexamethasone, a corticosteroid, along with supplementary oxygen can also help.

## High Altitude Retinal Hemorrhage

High altitude retinal hemorrhages occur when blood vessels in the brain burst. Although they can be unpleasant to look at—occasionally the entire sclera, the white portion of the eye, can be flooded with red blood—generally it's considered harmless, as vision is usually not affected.

If vision is affected, it should be viewed as a sign that you should climb no further and should begin descent. High altitude retinal hemorrhage with vision effects is considered a sign that HAPE or HACE will occur in the near future.

## DROWNING

Drowning happens when respiratory passages are blocked by liquid and you breathe in the liquid instead of air. It's most common in small children; babies can drown in as little as an inch of water. Contrary to Hollywood depictions of drowning as a dramatic struggle against the elements, drowning is typically—eerily—silent. It's also difficult to recognize drowning from a distance. What's known as the instinctive drowning response is an automatic set of behaviors triggered in the body by the sensation of suffocation in water, when a person is, or is very close to, drowning. These behaviors include lateral flapping, pressing one's arms in the water in an attempt to rise high enough to breathe, trying to roll over to one's back in an attempt to float, and tilting one's head back. It almost never entails screaming for help or waving one's arms.

## Performing CPR

- For an adult or child, put the heel of your hand in the center of the chest at the nipple line. For an infant, use two fingers on the breastbone.
- Press down two inches for an adult or child, making sure not to press down on the ribs; press down an inch and a half on an infant, making sure not to press down at the end of the breast bone.
- You're going to do thirty chest compressions at the rate of one hundred compressions a minute (roughly equal to the beat of the Bee Gees' "Stayin' Alive" or Queen's "Another One Bites the Dust"). Check to see if the person is breathing.
- If the patient is not breathing, you should pinch the nose to create a tight seal, breathe two puffs of air into the mouth, and repeat the chest compressions. Repeat until the person starts breathing or help arrives.

## Assisting Drowning Victims

If you find someone has drowned, the first step is to remove him or her from the water. Check to see if the person is breathing, either by placing your ear near the mouth and nose to see if you feel air on your cheek or by watching to see if the chest is rising. If the person is not breathing, check their pulse for ten seconds. If there's no pulse, you should commence cardio pulmonary resuscitation (CPR). If you haven't been trained in CPR, follow these basic instructions.

Drowning can be prevented by being incredibly vigilant with small children around bodies of water, learning how to swim, always swimming with a buddy, and avoiding water bodies with hazardous conditions such as strong rapids and rip tides.

## Dry Drowning

Just because you manage to successfully get someone breathing after a drowning doesn't mean the patient is out of the woods. Dry drowning, also known as secondary drowning, occurs when you breathe in water and your vocal chords spasm, closing off the airways and making it harder to breathe. This is most prevalent in children, though it can happen in adults, and symptoms include coughing, chest pain, trouble breathing, and feeling extremely tired. There's no set course of treatment—symptoms usually resolve themselves after twenty-four hours, but supplementary oxygen and a breathing tube may be necessary.

## INFECTIOUS DISEASES

### Lyme Disease

Lyme disease is named for the village of Old Lyme, Connecticut, where the condition was first identified. It is a bacterial infection spread by the bite of blacklegged ticks, most commonly the deer tick. Deer ticks are a reddish brown color, roughly a tenth of an inch, or the size of a ballpoint pen tip. In the United States it is most prevalent in the northeast, from Virginia through Maine and in Wisconsin.

#### Symptoms of Lyme Disease

Lyme disease patients may experience a small, red bump at the site of the tick bite, but such bumps are normal and not necessarily suggestive of the disease. If the redness expands to form a classic bull's-eye pattern, this is what is known as a signature of Lyme disease. You might develop the rash in several areas of the body and experience flu-like symptoms such as fever, chills, headache, and body aches. However, roughly 50 percent of people don't experience the bull's-eye pattern, which, in addition to the vagueness of symptoms, can lead to an under-reporting of the disease. Blood tests, or a test of the tick itself (if found), can confirm the presence of the disease.

### Treating Lyme Disease

Standard treatment is a course of antibiotics: oxycycline, amoxicillin, or cefuroxime axetil. Untreated or under-treated Lyme disease can cause some people to develop symptoms, including problems with the brain and nervous system, muscles and joints, heart and circulation, digestion, reproductive system, and skin, that linger weeks, months, or years after original infection which is called chronic Lyme disease. Medical treatment is necessary to help resolve it, or maintain symptoms.

### Preventing Infection

Ticks are active any time the temperature is above freezing, but the tick needs to be attached to your body for twenty-four hours for it to transmit disease-causing bacteria. Preventative measures include avoiding contact with ticks by avoiding wooded and brushy areas with high grass and leaf litter, as well as using repellents that contain 20 to 30 percent DEET on exposed skin and clothing, though care should be taken when applying DEET to children. Permethrin is an insect repellant that can be applied to clothing and provide protection through multiple washings (follow instructions on the bottle regarding application in ventilated areas, and allowing clothes to dry fully). Additionally, you should wear light-colored clothing, which makes tick identification easier.

When you return home, or every evening while camping, you should scan your body for any signs of ticks—have a partner look you over for any areas that are hard for you to examine yourself. If you find a tick, you should remove it by grasping the tick close to the skin with tweezers, pulling the tick straight out, and cleaning the skin with antiseptic. If possible, save the tick for later testing and see a doctor for diagnosis. If not possible, monitor the area for the classic rash, and be on guard for flu-like symptoms. Do not try to remove the tick by burning it off or using other folk remedies.

## Tick Paralysis

Tick paralysis is caused by a neurotoxin in the tick's saliva that is injected when the tick bites a person.

### Symptoms of Tick Paralysis

Symptoms, which begin as a weakness in both legs that progress to paralysis, begin two to seven days after a bite. It can also present as general lack of muscle coordination without muscle weakness. Left unchecked, however, the paralysis moves upwards to the torso, arms, and head, possibly leading to respiratory failure and death.

### Treatment of Tick Paralysis

In most cases, treatment is straightforward: find and remove the tick using tweezers, as described in the section on Lyme disease on pages 102-3. The patient will recover after a few days. However, in the case of the Australian paralysis tick, which is only found on the eastern coast of Australia, an anti-tick serum is needed or the paralysis will continue and lead to death.

## Malaria

Malaria is a mosquito-borne infection caused by a parasite that is most prevalent in tropical countries, particularly those of sub-Saharan Africa, South America, and Southeast Asia. Prior to the late twentieth century it was also prevalent in the American south (especially in Florida and Louisiana), but the pesticide DDT helped to eradicate it. With a warming climate and limited use of pesticides due to their health impacts on both humans and animals, there is some concern that tropical diseases are migrating north again.

### Symptoms of Malaria

Symptoms of malaria include chills, headache, sweats, fatigue, nausea, and vomiting that can cycle every forty-eight to seventy-two hours depending on the strain of malaria. (One strain, *P. falciparum*, does not cause a cyclic fever.) Symptoms can appear in as little as seven days or as long as eight to ten months after infection, with incubation lasting longer among those on anti-malarial medications or those with immunities due to prior infection.

### Treating Malaria

While some people are able to fight off malaria without treatment, they run the risk of the parasite-filled blood cells blocking the small blood vessels in their brains in what is known as cerebral malaria. The brain swells, and brain damage can occur causing coma and even death.

Active forms of the parasite are treated with a host of drugs including chloroquine, atovaquone-proguanil, artemether-lumefantrine, mefloquine, quinine (which is the tonic in tonic water but less than a therapeutic dose), quinidine, doxycycline (used in combination with quinine), and clindamycin (used in combination with quinine). Because some strains of malaria can "hide" in the liver and cause relapses weeks and months down the line, primaquine works to kill the dormant parasite liver forms but should not be taken by pregnant women or people deficient in G6PD (glucose-6-phosphate dehydrogenase). A screening test is necessary to determine if you're deficient in G6PD. All of the drugs require a prescription, though it is possible to buy cinchona bark, which contains quinine fairly easily, though below therapeutic doses.

### Preventing Infection

It's important to note that drug-resistant malaria is quite prevalent, and chloroquine-resistant malaria is found in all corners of the malaria world except for Central America, the Middle East, and Haiti and the Dominican Republic. Like Lyme disease, prevention is critical. Avoid going out between dusk and dawn, when mosquitoes are most likely to bite. Use repellants that contain DEET as detailed in the Lyme disease section, and sleep under pesticide-treated mosquito nets, making sure that you don't touch the nets in your sleep.

## Yellow Fever

Yellow fever is a viral hemorrhagic (bleeding) disease that, like malaria, is spread by mosquitoes. The virus incubates in the body for three to six days after infection. A blood test is necessary to definitively determine infection.

### Symptoms of Yellow Fever

Common symptoms include fever, chills, headache, muscle aches, nausea, loss of appetite, dizziness, and redness of the eyes, face, and tongue. Most patients improve after three to five days of illness. Fifteen percent of people enter a second, more toxic phase in which their skin becomes jaundiced (colored yellow due to liver damage) and there is bleeding from the mouth nose, eyes, or stomach. Blood appears in patients' vomit and feces, and kidney function falls drastically. Half of all people who enter this phase will die.

### Treatment and Prevention of Yellow Fever

Yellow fever is exceedingly common in the tropical areas of Africa and Latin America and has no known cure. Treatment is focused on reducing symptoms and improving patient comfort. It is a difficult disease to diagnose, because its symptoms—headache, backache, shivers, and fever—are similar to that of malaria, dengue fever, and viral hepatitis. Vaccination is the only way to avoid getting yellow fever; a single dose is enough to provide lifelong immunity.

## West Nile Virus

Like malaria, West Nile is a mosquito-borne virus. Unlike malaria, however, most people who are infected (70 to 80 percent) never show symptoms. One in five patients develop a fever, body aches, headaches, vomiting, joint pains, diarrhea, or rash. Managing symptoms, by giving fever-reducing medication and making sure the patient stays hydrated, is generally enough.

### Treatment of Severe West Nile Virus

Roughly 1 percent of patients (usually people over the age of sixty and individuals with compromised immune systems due to cancer, organ transplants, etc.) will develop encephalitis or viral meningitis. Symptoms include high fever, neck stiffness, disorientation, and coma. Hospitalization in these cases might be recommended, because they can get intravenous fluids and round-the-clock care and attention. Still, there's no cure for West Nile virus, and 10 percent of those who develop cerebral symptoms will die.

## *Prevention of West Nile Virus*

Prevention mirrors that of malaria prevention. Avoid being outside between dusk and dawn, use repellants, and sleep under mosquito nets in homes that don't have screens to keep mosquitoes out.

# Rabies

Rabies is a virus transmitted through the bite of a rabid animal; the virus is deposited into your muscle and fatty tissues and begins replicating. The easiest way to prevent rabies is to avoid getting bitten—don't approach strange, unfamiliar animals, and definitely don't try to pet them. In the United States, rabies is most often transmitted via the saliva of bats, coyotes, foxes, raccoons, and skunks. But even if you're familiar with an animal, avoid it if it's behaving unusually. If you are bitten, it's not always possible to determine if the animal is rabid (or just cranky). Rabid animals can appear asymptomatic.

## *Symptoms of Rabies*

Early symptoms mimic the flu (fever, aches, weakness, and general discomfort) and last anywhere from two to ten days. As the disease progresses it begins to impact the brain: hallucinations, delirium, insomnia, and manic behavior develop in what is known as furious rabies. In a less common form of rabies, paralytic rabies, the muscles slowly stop working and the patient slips into a coma and dies.

## *Treating Rabies Infections*

A treatment called human rabies immune globulin (HRIG) can be administered the day of the bite, and five shots of the rabies vaccine is then given over twenty-eight days. The rabies vaccine can also be taken as a preventative measure, especially among those (spelunkers, rabies researchers, veterinarians) at a high risk for infection. After the initial shot, a second shot is administered a year later, and a booster shot every three to five years.

Once a person shows symptoms of rabies, treatment is no longer effective and the disease is fatal.

# Tapeworm

A tapeworm is a kind of parasitic flatworm that usually infects the digestive tract. Tapeworm infections happen after eating unwashed (usually uncooked) foods that are contaminated with tapeworm eggs, eating undercooked meat from contaminated animals, or drinking from a tainted water source.

### Signs and Symptoms

Most people with an intestinal tapeworm infection have no symptoms, though some people have upper abdominal discomforts, diarrhea, and a loss of appetite. Anemia in people with a fish tapeworm is also possible. The easiest way to diagnose a tapeworm infection is by looking at your stool: infected people will periodically pass segments of the parasite (that look like white worms) in their stool. Occasionally tapeworms can migrate to the brain, causing headaches, seizures, and other brain issues, but an MRI is needed to make a diagnosis.

### Treating and Preventing Tapeworms

Treatment is an oral medication call praziquantel. Tapeworms can be avoided by refraining from eating raw fish and meat, thoroughly cooking meat, washing hands before cooking, and refraining from eating raw fruits and vegetables from countries where tapeworm is a problem.

## Typhoid Fever

Typhoid fever is a human-borne disease in which the *Salmonella typhi* bacteria is spread from person to person. While most people infected with *Salmonella typhi* bacteria are symptomatic, some people (like the infamous Typhoid Mary) can carry the infection without showing symptoms of the disease. Typhoid is most prevalent in parts of the world where clean water (and thus handwashing) is scarce.

### Symptoms of Typhoid

Symptoms of typhoid fever include a sustained high fever—as high as 103°F–104°F—weakness, stomach pains, loss of appetite, and headache. Some patients develop a rash of flat, rose-colored spots, though the only way to definitively diagnose typhoid fever is by testing blood or stool samples. Diarrhea or constipation is also common.

### Treating and Preventing Typhoid

Certain antibiotics, usually ciprofloxacin or ceftriaxone, can clear up the infection. While sick with fever and diarrhea, it is very important for the patient to drink a lot of fluids.

There are two ways to avoid typhoid fever. One is to avoid eating risky foods and drinks (e.g., foods unlikely to have been prepared in sanitary conditions). Only drink boiled or bottled water (if bottled, make sure the seal is intact), eat foods that are hot and served still steaming, and only eat raw fruits and vegetables that you can peel yourself (after washing your hands in clean water) or avoid them altogether. Getting vaccinated is also important. Vaccinations last for several years before requiring a booster.

## Tetanus

Tetanus, also known as lockjaw, is a serious bacterial infection that affects the nervous system, leading to extremely painful muscle contractions. It is caused by a bacteria present in soil, animal feces, and dust and usually enters the body through a wound (the iconic rusty nail, as well as splinters). Tetanus can also form through crush injuries, tattoos, animal bites, and even ear infections. Once infected it can take anywhere from a few days to a few months to show symptoms, but the average incubation time is seven to twelve days.

### Symptoms of Tetanus

Symptoms include spasms and stiffness in the jaw muscles (hence the name lockjaw), stiffness in neck muscles, and painful body spasms triggered by a draft, a loud noise, physical touch, or even light. Since tetanus affects the body's muscles, the patient may experience difficulty breathing, which can become life-threatening.

### Treating Tetanus

There's no cure for tetanus, and medical attention rests on managing symptoms. The best way to avoid tetanus, however, is by getting vaccinated (once every ten years) and getting a booster shot immediately after suffering an injury that is likely to put you at risk of contracting tetanus.

## Meningitis

Meningitis occurs when the protective membranes that cover your brain and spinal cord, known as the meninges, become inflamed. Although meningitis can be caused by a physical injury, cancer, or even certain drugs, the most common causes of meningitis are bacterial and viral.

## *Bacterial Meningitis*

Roughly 80 percent of all cases of acute meningitis are bacterial meningitis, and children are particularly at risk. Symptoms include high fever, headaches, and neck stiffness that make it difficult to lower your chin to your chest. The good news is that it can be treated successfully with antibiotics. The most common antibiotics prescribed are: ampicillin, cefotaxime, ceftriaxone, gentamicin, penicillin G, rifampin, and vancomycin (though vancomycin is generally only used as an antibiotic when the infection has proven resistant to other ones). Unfortunately, the antibiotics work best when given intravenously, usually with a corticosteroid to reduce the inflammation. Ten percent of people who contract bacterial meningitis die, but if treated early, most people recover. Absent treatment, or absent rapid treatment, if the patient survives, he or she may endure lifelong paralysis, seizures, and mental impairment. The best form of prevention is getting vaccinated—the meningitis vaccine protects against most strains.

## *Viral Meningitis*

Unlike bacterial meningitis, viral meningitis is generally not life-threatening. Treatment generally consists of supporting the patient's wellbeing: rest, plenty of fluids, and pain- and fever-reducing medications like acetaminophen and ibuprofen are prescribed as needed. The biggest difficulty with viral meningitis is delineating it from bacterial, absent medical testing. Generally, if the person's condition deteriorates rapidly, assume it's bacterial.

# CHAPTER 6

## WHOLE BODY MAINTENANCE

### HEALING AND TREATING TOPICAL WOUNDS AND UNCOMFORTABLE AILMENTS

### Assessment of Injuries

When you or someone you know gets injured, the default is to do something, *anything*. But looking before you leap can cause more harm than good. If, for example, you move someone with a spinal injury without first immobilizing them, you can cause permanent paralysis. You can also miss key clues as to how to treat their injuries before they get worse.

### Identifying the Situation

When you arrive on a scene where someone is injured, the first thing you should do is follow the three Cs of first aid: Check, Call, and Care. First, check for injuries using the mnemonic "DR. ABC."

---

### DR. ABC

Danger: Are you and the patient safe? Is there a bear lurking in the corners?

Response: Is the patient awake and responsive? If not, call EMS and then check their ABC.

Airway: Make sure nothing is blocking the patient's airway. If clear, move on. If blocked, facilitate the opening of the airway. In conscious patients, try to remove any obstruction, perhaps by using abdominal thrusts (see page 171). In unconscious patients, tilt the head to lift the chin and hopefully open the airway. Once airway is open, move on.

---

*(Continued on next page)*

| | |
|---|---|
| Breathing: | Is the person breathing normally? If not, you need to call EMS (if you haven't already) and then perform assistance. You can help a conscious person in removing any blockage. If the patient's unconscious and not breathing, attempt CPR (see pages 172-173).). Don't move onto the next step until they're breathing. |
| Circulation: | Is there a pulse? Is the patient bleeding heavily? Treat sites of severe bleeding to prevent shock. |

Once a basic assessment is completed, call for emergency medical services. You need to call for EMS as soon as you assess that a person is in need of real medical attention and BEFORE you begin providing care. If you're with another person, have that person call for emergency services while you begin to care for the person's injuries.

## Spinal Injuries

If you suspect a spinal injury, take care not to move the patient and immobilize the head and neck if possible. Symptoms of a spinal injury include extreme back pain or pressure in the person's neck, head, or back. Additional symptoms include: weakness or paralysis in the body; a loss of sensation in hands, fingers, feet, or toes; loss of control over bladder and bowel (if the person urinates or defecates themselves without noticing); difficulty walking due to balance problems; impaired breathing (effortful breathing with no physical obstruction); and odd body position such as a twisted neck or back.

## Recovery Position

If a person is unconscious but breathing and has no other pressing, life-threatening conditions, you should put them in the recovery position. In the recovery position, the patient is prone on their side, with arms and legs positioned to help with balance. The recovery position helps ensure that airways will remain open, since choking on vomit or their own saliva is less likely.

112

## Steps to Putting Someone in the Recovery Position

- Kneel on the floor to one side of the person.
- Take the arm nearest to you and place it so that it's outstretched, parallel to the body from the shoulder to the elbow. Bend the arm at the elbow so the hand is pointed upwards towards the head and the arm itself looks like a backward L. This keeps the arm out of the way for when you roll the person over.
- Take the other hand, stretch it across the person's body, and tuck it under the opposite cheek like a small child falling asleep. The back of the hand should be touching the cheek.
- Take the knee farthest from you and bend it into a right angle. Roll the person onto his or her side by pulling on the bent knee. The bent knee should be resting on top of the other, straight leg. The top arm (the one you tucked under the cheek) supports the head, while the bottom arm will stop you from over-rolling the person.
- Open the patient's airway by carefully tilting the head back and checking for obstructions.
- Stay with the person, monitoring his or her pulse until help arrives.
- If the injuries will allow you to, turn the person onto the other side after thirty minutes, but place in the same rescue position.

## Treating Bleeding

If an adult loses more than two pints of blood, or a child loses three-quarters of a pint of blood, they can go into shock or even die. When faced with someone who is bleeding, your goal is to stop the bleeding, and make sure that the wound is clean and properly bandaged (more details on page 120). If bleeding is severe, you also want to treat the person for shock (see pages 167-168). Seek attention from a medical expert as soon as possible.

### Treating Bleeding from Superficial Wounds

Superficial wounds just affect the top few layers of the skin. They are the kind we associate with the bumps and scrapes of everyday living.

Blood tends to ooze or creep out of superficial wounds, which makes treating them relatively easy and straightforward. Wash the wound with soap and water. Although rubbing alcohol or hydrogen peroxide are commonly used, they can actually inhibit wound healing and should be avoided.

### Treating Bleeding from Serious Wounds

More serious wounds require more care. First, lay the person down, because blood loss at this level can make them faint, especially if the person is standing upright. Laying them down reduces this risk by increasing blood flow to the brain. If possible, elevate the body part that is bleeding.

Remove any dirt or debris that you can see in the wound. If the wound is the result of an object—a knife, arrow, stick, piece of pipe—DO NOT remove the object, as it can cause additional damage or make the bleeding worse. Instead place pads and bandages around the object and tape the object into place.

If there is no object in the wound, place pressure on the wound directly using a bandage, cloth, or clothing. The cleaner the fabric you're using, the better. You want to reduce the risk of infection. If there's nothing available, use your hand (preferably while wearing a medical glove). Maintain pressure until the bleeding stops. Once it has stopped, gently clean the wound using water, saline, and Betadine (povidone-iodine). The wound may start bleeding again slightly—that's normal. Dress the wound with bandage, tape, or a piece of clothing, and place a cold pack over the area. If bleeding continues, don't remove the bandage; you want to maintain pressure, so just place a new cloth over the old one.

## SKIN INJURIES

Oft-forgotten, skin is the largest organ in the human body. This super elastic organ helps us regulate body temperature, maintain the right amount of water in the body, and keep out a large number of harmful germs while providing our organs the space they need to function. Here are some common maladies that can strike the skin.

## Wounds

Wounds are injuries to the body's living tissue (often the skin) caused by cuts, blows or other physical trauma. A haircut isn't a wound because your hair isn't alive, but a paper cut is a wound, albeit a small one.

Your first step when dealing with a wound is to assess the situation. Determine if the wound is life-threatening. Some examples include wounds where bodily organs (in addition to the skin) are involved, like a puncture wound to the stomach. How old is the wound? Is it fresh, i.e., less than six hours old? Or is it much older—perhaps weeks—and for some reason not healing? What's the source of the wound? Animal bites for example, might require rabies shots, and the wounds need to be more carefully cleansed because animal saliva can carry a range of infectious organisms. A small foot injury that refuses to heal might be the cause of an underlying issue like poor circulation or diabetes that also needs to be addressed.

### Treating Wounds

The basics of wound care can be distilled into three simple maxims: keep it clean, keep it moist, and keep it nourished.

Remove any debris from the injury; rocks, dirt, and twigs that remain in the wound can be a source of injury. Then use soap and fresh water, preferably flowing either from a clean bottle or a faucet, to gently cleanse and rinse the wound.

Cover the wound with petroleum jelly or a wound ointment and a bandage to keep it moist. While antibacterial ointments were once heavily encouraged, an increasing awareness of antibiotic resistance suggests that their routine use should be discouraged. Most cuts and wounds will heal perfectly fine without them. If the cut was unusually dirty, however, it's fine to use an antibacterial. An alternative to antibacterial ointments is honey. Used for millennia on wounds and burns, honey both keeps the wound moist and has natural antimicrobial properties that inhibit infection. Many drugstores now stock medical grade honey for its specific use in wound care.

Keep it nourished by not bandaging your wound with so much pressure that it blocks off blood flow. A little bit of pressure when a wound initially forms can help stop excessive bleeding until your body has time to clot the wound itself. Once the wound has stopped bleeding, however, you want blood to flow since it brings the nourishment necessary for the wound to heal. Use enough pressure to keep the bandage in place, but not so much that you inhibit blood flow to the area.

## Abrasions

Abrasions are wounds that cause damage that is only skin deep. Minor abrasions may tear up the skin a bit, but they generally don't bleed or scar. Deeper abrasions or ones on thin-skinned, bony areas (like knees and ankles) are more prone to bleeding and scarring. Either way, skin abrasions may hurt a bit, but they're not life-threatening. To treat, wash the abrasion with soap and water, gently removing any dirt or debris in the wound. Cover the abrasion with a bandage for roughly five days. This will protect it from dirt, while the moisture will speed healing. You should change the bandage daily. For cuts and scrapes that are hard to keep clean, use Betadine, an iodine-based antiseptic. Forget peroxide and rubbing alcohol, which can actually slow healing.

## Puncture Wounds

Puncture wounds are stab wounds, whether they come from stepping on a nail or from a splinter. To treat a puncture wound, remove the object that caused the puncture as long as it's small and not hitting any vital organs. Every so often, you'll hear stories of someone accidentally sending a nail gun flying into their skull—that is not a puncture wound you should attempt to treat yourself.

Because of their incredibly small size, splinters in particular are very difficult to remove. The conventional method involves sterilizing a needle and using it to slip under the splinter to lift it closer to the surface of the skin. An alternative approach that many have found successful (if a bit more time consuming) is to make a poultice out of Epsom salt on a bandage and wrap it around the finger, changing it once or twice a day so it remains moist. After a day or two, the splinter will move towards the surface of the skin where it can easily be pulled out with a tweezer.

Once the item is out, rinse the wound under clean water for several minutes. If the wound is still bleeding, stop the bleeding by applying pressure with a clean cloth until the bleeding stops. Because puncture wounds involve an unclean item in your body, the risk for infection is higher than, say, for an abrasion. You don't want to stop the bleeding immediately, assuming it's a relatively small amount, because you want your body to clear some of the debris from the wound if possible. After stopping the bleeding, apply iodine and an antibacterial ointment, and bandage the wound. If you haven't had a tetanus shot in recent years, you should get a booster.

## Fishhook Wounds

These injuries are a unique type of a puncture. They are often incredibly dirty from the presence of marine bacteria, and the hook itself is difficult to remove because of barbs that stick in the skin. Removing the fishhook is best done by a medical professional, but doctors can be scarce when you're out on a fishing boat.

Don't attempt to remove fishhooks from vital or sensitive organs (like your eye). If you get a fishhook in your eye, remove it from the line, place a cup over your eye, and cover up the other eye as well (to minimize movement). These techniques also assume that you either have a high threshold for pain or are using some form of a local anesthetic. Finally, regular rules about cleaning and bandaging a puncture wound still apply here (if not doubly so).

### The Retrograde Technique

This works well on a barbless fishhook that is not deeply embedded. You apply downward pressure to the shank of the hook which helps to disengage the barb. The hook can then be backed out of the skin along the same path that it entered the body. If you feel resistance or the barb catching, you should stop and try another removal method.

### The String-Yank Technique

Loop a string such as fishing line along the middle of the bend in the hook as you press down on the shank of the fishhook; pull upward quickly and firmly on the string.

### The Advance and Cut Technique

This works best when the point of the fish hook is already located near the surface of the skin. In that case, work to advance the hook forward, closer to the surface. Once the barb surfaces, cut the barb off using pliers or some other tool, freeing you to slip the rest of the hook out via the path it used to enter.

## Scalp Wounds

Scalp wounds are unusually bloody because the face and scalp have more blood vessels close to the surface than other parts of the body. If the skull is deformed (there are sunken areas, bone is visible, or worse, parts of the brain are visible), or the injury involves the eye, you should seek immediate medical attention. Have the person lie down, remove any visible objects from the wound, and then press down on the wound with gauze or a clean cloth for fifteen minutes without peeking at the wound first. Every time you remove pressure "just to check," you delay clotting. If blood soaks through your cloth, apply another one without lifting the first. After fifteen minutes most head wounds will have stopped bleeding or slowed to a trickle. If bleeding has stopped, you can stop applying pressure; if bleeding has not ceased, call for help. While applying pressure, look for signs of shock (such as loss of consciousness—more details on pages 167-168). Once the wound has fully stopped bleeding, follow the steps of basic wound care.

## Wound Closure

Most wounds will close and heal on their own. In some cases, especially when the wound is larger than three-quarters of an inch or reaches down to tissue or bone, it's beneficial to use mechanical ways of closing the wound. This can reduce scarring (especially in the case of facial wounds) or speed healing. The pressure of suturing (better known as stitching), gluing, or taping wounds closed will stop bleeding and prevent infection.

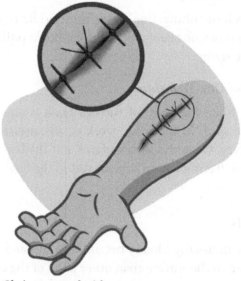

*Closing a wound with sutures.*

### Sutures

Suturing involves a needle (straight, circular, or curved) and thread, which can be made from several different materials, commonly including nylon, polyester, and polypropylene. Some sutures contain an antimicrobial coating designed to reduce the likelihood of infection.

Traditionally, after the wound healed, sutures needed to be removed, but a number of absorbable sutures now exist where the body breaks down the thread material over time and the sutures don't have to be removed. Which needle and thread is used depends on the area of the body being stitched and the type of wound. Sutures have to be strong enough to securely hold the tissue in place, but flexible enough to be stitched and withstand movement of the body after stitching. They also can't trigger allergies, and they can't be absorbent or else they'd allow fluids and infection to enter the body along the suture line.

Sutures should be cleansed daily and kept dry. In the case of scalp sutures, hair should be washed every two days with a gentle shampoo; hair products should be avoided until the wound heals, as should activities that stretch the skin around the suture. While some bleeding from sutures is normal, especially when the sutures are fresh and you've just cleaned them, excessive bleeding (enough to bleed through a bandage, for example) is not normal and you should seek immediate medical attention. Similarly, if the wound begins to hurt more, it starts to smell, a fever develops, or the wound feels hot to the touch, seek additional attention—it's a sign that the wound might be infected.

### Skin Glue

Like sutures, skin glue is used to bring skin together. However, while suturing requires stitching and local anesthesia, skin glue requires neither. It is less effective and less durable than stitching on large wounds, but is very effective for wounds up to two inches long with straight edges that need temporary stabilization. It can also be used at the edges of stitches, or over stitches.

The glue used by medical professionals is slightly different from the typical superglue available at the store. Dermabond is such a medical glue used by and available to professionals, but liquid bandage products, such as New-Skin, are readily available at drug stores. Veterinary glues are also commercially available, although they are not officially approved for use on humans.

## Surgical Stapling

Staples are used for similar reasons to suturing, but staples are faster. These aren't your regular office staplers, but sterilized medical-grade machines that are most commonly used in surgical settings. Staples have to be removed as the wound heals.

# Wound Dressings

Dressings come in a variety of shapes and sizes. The best wound dressing or covering depends on the type, size, and location of the injury. As a rule of thumb, the best dressings provide a clean, moist environment for the wound, enabling it to heal without sticking to it or causing additional injury.

## Butterfly Bandages

Butterfly bandages are good for wounds that are short but deep. They help to close the gap, reducing scarring, and speeding healing, in much the same way that wound glue is used. Wound glue however also helps the wound maintain moisture.

## Adhesive Bandages

Adhesive bandages stick to the skin and are most frequently used in a home setting. They come in a variety of shapes and sizes and usually consist of a sterile pad stuck to an adhesive strip.

## Sterile Pads

Sterile pads are thin pieces of cloth-like material that can be used to protect wounds from bacteria and other infections. Because they're sterile, they won't introduce new infection to the wound. And because they don't have adhesive, you can stack and fold them in ways that you couldn't with an adhesive bandage. They are usually used in conjunction with gauze or tape to hold them in place.

## Gauze

Gauze is a thin, loosely woven, cotton-like material used for wrapping wounds and large body parts and for keeping sterile pads in place. They're beneficial because they wrap around the body, and they can provide additional support and pressure if necessary. Stretch gauze in particular is very good at providing support.

*Sterile Burn Sheets*

Burn sheets are made of special laminated tissue fibers that cover a burn without sticking it to burn the way that bandages and sterile pads frequently do.

## Mouth and Tongue Lacerations

These lacerations are painful because we use our tongues and mouths so much. If the tongue laceration only goes partway through the mouth, you can treat it at home; doctors will avoid stitching tongue injuries unless they're very deep. After making sure that whatever caused the laceration is removed, an ice cube wrapped in a thin cloth and then applied to the wound for one to three minutes six to ten times on the day of the injury can help with pain and swelling. Rinse the mouth with a warm saltwater wash four to six times for the first few days, and maintain good oral hygiene, including use of an antiseptic mouth wash. Finally, give the tongue a break and stick to soft foods. Over-the-counter pain medications can also provide some assistance.

Blisters are small bubbles filled with fluid that form on the skin due to friction, burning or other damage. If the blister doesn't hurt too much, the best bet is to keep it intact where the skin provides a barrier against infection, and simply cover it with tape. If the blister hurts too much, you can drain it while keeping the skin intact. After washing your hands and the blister with soap and water, swab the blister with iodine or rubbing alcohol. Sterilize a clean, sharp needle using alcohol. Then, using the sterilized needle makes a few small puncture holes near the edge of the blister. Let the fluid drain but leave the skin in place. Cover the blister with an antibacterial ointment and change the dressing. Friction blisters can usually be avoided by wearing properly fitting clothes and other garments.

## Burns
### Thermal Burns

Thermal burns are cause by an external heat source, ranging from a hot pot on the oven to an open flame. The type of burn and its severity dictates your course of treatment, but never apply butter or oils to a burn.

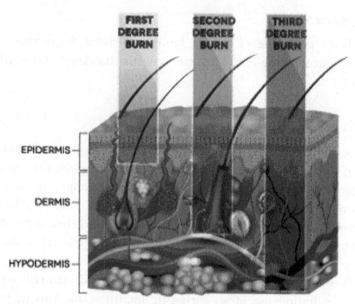

*Damage caused by first-, second-, and third-degree burns.*

## First-Degree Burns

First-degree burns only involve the outermost layer of the skin, similar to a case of mild sunburn. The skin turns red, but is white to the touch and painful.

To treat a first-degree burn, extricate yourself from the source of the burn. Hold the burned skin under cool water until pain subsides. Then, as in sunburn, aloe vera gel can be applied to help soothe the burn after the area has cooled.

## Second-Degree Burns

Second-degree burns involve the epidermis and some portion of the dermis (the second layer of the skin). Like first-degree burns, the skin becomes red and turns white to the touch. However, blisters form in second-degree burns and they may not be painful because nerve endings might have been destroyed. This burn may or may not require medical attention. If the blister is less than two inches, or doesn't ooze, it is likely fine to treat yourself.

Rinse the burn with cool water to stop the pain, then clean the burn area with mild soap and water making sure not to break the blisters.

Some skin may come off while treating. Apply an ointment; there are a growing number of honey-based ointments on the market that have been shown to be as, if not more, effective than other dressings for moderate burns. Bandage the burn using a burn dressing; traditional bandages can stick to burns, re-injuring the area and delaying healing.

### Third-Degree Burns

Third-degree burns are the most severe involving all layers of the skin and potentially affecting muscle and bone. Nerve endings and sweat glands are all destroyed; skin may look leathery, charred, and dried. This burn absolutely requires medical attention. Use cool compresses to sooth the areas while you rush the person to medical help or help comes to you.

## EYES

The eyes are often said to be the windows to the soul. In more practical terms, they show us the beauty of the world around us and the practicality of being able to function within the world. It's important that we take good care of them.

## Caring for Contact Lenses and Homemade Saline Solution

In a perfect world, we would all have perfect vision. This is not the case, and if you happen to be a contact lens wearer, there are few discomforts greater than having dried out, torn, or otherwise damaged contacts as your only option for managing and maintaining clear vision. Commercially sold contact solution should be your primary resource for lens cleansing. It is not recommended to make homemade contact solution for extended use, but when you are away from modern conveniences and uncertain of how long you have between now and your next opportunity to replenish your stockpile, you may have to resort to brewing up your own in a pinch.

### Removing Stuck Lenses

When you are away from modern conveniences or the comforts of regular hygiene, maintaining good eye health can feel like a nuisance, but it is still vitally important. When you have fewer opportunities to remove and clean your lenses, they are more likely to get stuck. If this is the case, you should remain calm and remember that eyes are closed pockets; your lost, folded, stuck, or ripped lens can move around, but it can't truly get lost. Always wash your hands with a non-cream soap and warm water before touching your eyes or handling contact lenses. With one hand, use your clean thumb and forefinger to move your lid away from your eye. Locate the missing lens, which will likely still have a light hue to distinguish it from your eye. Gently nudge the lens, moistening it with contact solution if necessary. If the lens is not causing severe pain, you can let it sit in your eye for twenty minutes or so and see if it moves to a more workable spot on its own. If your lens is causing even more trouble and cannot be moved gently with your fingertips, you may need to use a contact lens plunger. These are small devices that attach to the lens and use light suction to pull the lens away from your eye.

## Storage

Always store contacts in sterile, sealable cases. Never, under ANY circumstances, should you store your contacts in regular tap water. Tap water has bacteria, microbes, and even parasites in it, which have been known to cause unsightly and excruciating eye problems, and eventually even blindness. The same goes for leaving your contacts in for too long—never, ever do this! Leaving contact lenses in your eyes is the equivalent of suffocating your eye. It can lead to infection, and the lenses themselves will become dirty, dry, and harder to remove the longer they stay in.

## Homemade Contact Solution

At the most basic level, you can store your contact lenses in a sterile case with distilled water. Water that has been distilled has been condensed and freed of impurities, viruses, and bacteria, so you will not be at risk of damage to your eye. However, this is not ideal; using water to store your lenses can distort them. Without the added salinity, your contacts will absorb the water, change the shape, and even shrink the lens so that it molds improperly to your eye. The changes in shape can propel faster deterioration and eventual damage to the lenses.

To make your own contact solution, start with distilled water and sodium chloride. If you do not have sodium chloride, regular kitchen salt will work. Mix one teaspoon of salt for every liter or quart of distilled water.

Boil the water until the salt is properly dissolved and you have your solution. Store the saline solution in sterile containers, such as glass bottles with sealable tops that you have sanitized in boiling water. Seal the solution tightly and store it in a cool, dark place so that bacteria cannot grow. Prepare fresh solution each day and make sure to sanitize the containers between each use.

## Eye Patches

Eye patches and bandages are commonly recommended treatments for eye injuries. Children may also be required to wear an eye patch to balance out a weak or lazy eye, and when this occurs, the dominant eye is covered to strengthen the weak eye. The key thing to understand when patching an eye is that when we're awake, our default is to keep our eyes open; we struggle to keep them closed. Patching an eye should facilitate keeping the eye in the closed position. Because most eye patches don't directly contact the eye, you should put gauze over the closed eye first to create a very small amount of pressure before placing the eye patch over the socket. With the eye patch in place, you can use medical tape to affix the pad to the face. Place the tape along the outside edge of the patch, pressing down lightly for some, but not too much, pressure. Move upward across the eyebrow and downward across the cheek in a diagonal fashion. Some people prefer to eschew the use of tape and instead hold the sterile eye pad in place with a large bandage.

## Eye Irritants

When a foreign body, like sand, gets into an eye, the temptation is to rub the eye; the itching sensation can be almost unbearable. However, rubbing an eye when there's sand, grit, or other substances present can make the situation much worse. You risk scratching your cornea, irritating your eyelid, or spreading around chemical irritants. Instead, carefully treat each situation as described in the following sections.

### Minor Irritants in the Eye

In the case of eyelashes, sand, or glitter, the eyes will ordinarily remove these objects on their own through blinking and tearing. If they don't, wash hands thoroughly, remove contact lens if wearing one, and rinse the eye.

## Eye Rinse

Use an eye cup or another small cup, like a shot glass, filled with clean, lukewarm water. Lean forward and press the cup to your closed eye, creating a tight seal around your eye socket. Tilt your head backward, open your eye, and rotate your eyeball around so that the water is fully flushing your eye. Lean forward and remove the cup. The object may have been flushed out by now, but you may need to attempt this two or three times before the item is rinsed clear. If that doesn't work, or the object is embedded in your eyelid (not your eye), you can try using a moist cotton swab to lift it out, *making sure not to touch the eyeball.* If none of these work, there's a reasonable chance that the object is embedded in your eye and needs to be removed by a doctor.

## Foreign Objects in the Eye

When objects are embedded in the eye (shards of glass, for example), it's too sensitive a procedure for you to do yourself. You need to bandage *both* eyes, because the eyes are connected—where one goes the other follows. The only way to immobilize the injured eye is to bandage both eyes. Seek immediate medical attention.

## Chemicals in the Eye

When chemicals enter the eye, you must rinse your eyes immediately. The first ten to fifteen seconds are critical. To properly rinse your eyes, turn your head so the injured eye is down and to the side, hold your eyelids open, and flush with cool, clean, running water for at least five minutes for mildly irritating chemicals, twenty minutes for severe to moderate irritates and non-penetrating corrosives, and an hour for penetrating corrosives like lye. If a chemical eyewash station is present, use that instead; it will be easier to correctly position your body. If your contacts have not come out in the wash, attempt to remove them after rinsing. If they don't come out, don't force them. They may have adhered to your cornea. Seek medical help right away while continuing to flush your eyes with water or saline.

# Removing Contact Lenses

When you are prescribed contact lenses, your eye doctor should instruct you on how to properly insert and remove them. Regardless of contact type, the first step is always to wash your hands. There are numerous germs and bacteria that reside on your hand that can thrive in your eyes' warm, damp environment.

To remove soft contact lenses, look up and pull the lower lid down with the middle or ring finger of your dominant hand – the hand you use to write. Take your index finger and gently place it on the lower edge of your contact lens, sliding it to the whites of your eyes. You're doing it correctly if your vision will become less clear. Now, keeping your middle finger and index finger in place, squeeze the lens in between your index finger and thumb (they may gently graze your lower eyelid) and remove. Sometimes when your eye becomes too dry, soft contacts can fold and get "stuck" under your eye socket beyond the curve of the eyeball. Don't panic. Closing the eyelid for a while and then resuming "normal" eye behavior will eventually coax the contact lens out of its hiding place.

Hard contact lenses are removed by a different process. Cup your opposite hand under your eye (right hand under left eye, left hand under right eye). Looking down at your hand, place your index finger alongside the edge of your eye and remove the lens. You can also use a miniature plunger that uses suction to remove the contact lens.

## Corneal Abrasion

The cornea is the thin, clear, protective covering over your iris (the colored part of the eye) and the pupil (the small hole in your eye that expands and contracts in response to the amount of light in your environment). A corneal abrasion is a scratch on your cornea. Corneal abrasions can happen when something like a piece of sand or dirt gets into your eye, and you rub the eye in an attempt to get it out. Sometimes people with long nails accidentally scratch their cornea when inserting or removing contacts. Similarly, if you don't keep your contacts clean, or if you aggressively rub your eyes (such as during allergy season), you're risking a corneal abrasion. A symptom of a corneal abrasion is eye pain when exposed to bright light; the muscles surrounding the eye spasm so you have to squint. Sometimes people feel like there's something in their eye that they can't seem to get out.

Luckily, the discomfort associated with corneal abrasions is usually temporary. Corneal abrasions will usually heal on their own within one to three days. While the eye is healing, don't wear contacts or rub your eyes. *Do* wear sunglasses to protect your eyes against the sun's glare. Rinse eye with clean water if you find it soothing. If the pain is very severe, you might consider patching the eye, which helps with symptoms but not healing. You shouldn't do this if you're at a high risk for infection however, because you're reducing the amount of oxygen that your eye receives, making it more conducive to bacterial, fungal, and viral growth. If you wear contacts or if the abrasion was caused by contact with items that harbor bacteria and germs (vegetables, for example), you're at high risk for infection and shouldn't use an eye patch. Bandage contact lenses (different from corrective or cosmetic lenses) might also be recommended.

## Blunt Trauma

Blunt Trauma to the eye often occurs as a punch or a ball to the face. The two most common, striking examples of blunt trauma to the eye are the classic black eye and a bloody sclera (whites of the eye) known as a subconjunctival hemorrhage. While dramatic in appearance, these injuries are benign and heal themselves over the course of a few weeks. The best treatment for a black eye is to reduce swelling, while subconjunctival hemorrhages require no treatment.

However, an injury that is strong enough to cause a black eye or sub-conjunctival hemorrhage may also be severe enough to cause traumatic iritis. Traumatic iritis is an inflammation of the iris, or colored part of the eye that—if left untreated—can cause permanent damage and even blindness. Treatment can include steroids and cycloplegics, a type of drug that temporarily paralyses the injured eye to allow for healing while retaining use of the uninjured eye. Even with treatment, you'll likely suffer from some loss of vision. Additionally, there could be bleeding behind the eye in the space between the cornea and the iris, known as hyphemia, or a fracture of the eye socket. All of these require medical attention, which is why you should absolutely see a doctor after serious blunt force trauma to the eye.

## Photokeratitis

Also known as ultraviolet or snow blindness, photokeratitis happens when you stare directly at the sun, damaging your cornea. It's similar to a sunburn on the eye. Direct sunlight is not the only cause of photoker-atitis; sunlight reflected off snow, water, or ice, as well as some artificial sources of light like halogen lamps, tanning beds, and a welder's arc, can also cause photokeratitis. Like sunburn, we only sense damage once it's already done. Symptoms include a gritty feeling in the eye without any debris actually being present, pain, redness, tearing, and, very rarely, temporary vision loss. The upside is that photokeratitis usually goes away on its own, so treatment is primarily focused on soothing symptoms. Avoid wearing contacts, as they can irritate the eyes and slow healing. Get out of the sun and minimize sun exposure.

Prevention in this case is straightforward: wear UV-rated sunglasses when going outside, especially when it's sunny. In snow conditions, especially at higher elevations, it's possible to get photokeratitis even on cloudy days because the air is thinner and allows more UV rays to get through. If you do a lot of snowmobiling or mountaineering, there are clear or lighter colored lenses that still provide UV protection without darkening your vision. If you're a welder, wear suitable eye protection.

## Conjunctivitis

Better known as pink eye, conjunctivitis is an inflammation of the conjunctiva, the thin clear tissue that covers the white part of the eye and coats the inside of the eyelid. As the common name suggests, pink eye turns the tissues of the eye slightly pink. Additional symptoms include a thick yellow discharge that crusts over the eye (especially after sleeping), green or white discharge, blurred vision, and sensitivity to light. Pink eye can be caused by a bacterial infection, a viral infection (usually the same virus that causes the common cold), seasonal allergies, and irritants.

If the pink eye is caused by irritants, rinse the eyes with cool water; in the case of alkaline irritants like bleach, rinse with a lot of water and contact a doctor. If the pink eye is caused by allergies, dealing with the allergies by taking an antihistamine or other medications will alleviate the symptoms. Viral pink eye resolves itself within ten days, much like the common cold. Bacterial pink eye must be treated with antibiotics, in the form of pills or eye drops, prescribed by a physician. If pink eye appears in infants or babies, seek medical attention immediately, as it may be a sign of a more severe, eye-threatening infection.

## Sties

Sties are the sometimes painful, pimple-like bumps that appear along the edge of the eyelid. They're caused when an oil gland along the edge of the eyelid becomes infected by *Staphylococcus* bacteria. Usually we infect ourselves;

staphylococcal bacteria like to hang out in our nose, and if we rub our nose and then our eyes, we can pass the infection along. Fortunately, sties, while irritating, tend to clear up on their own after a few days, though a warm compress applied to the sty twice a day (morning and night) can help reduce inflammation and speed healing. You should never pop a sty, and avoid touching it. If you do touch it, make sure to wash your hands afterward; you don't want to spread the bacteria around—it is very contagious.

# NOSE

The nose is the gateway to the lungs. It provides our body with the air necessary for performing the functions that keep us alive. At the same time, it acts as the gatekeeper of infection, filtering out the worst pollutants, clueing us into harmful environments through smell, and making food worth eating—many of our sensory clues around how a food tastes are really based on how a food smells. This is partly why when you have a cold, food tastes less delicious; you can't really smell what you're eating.

## Nasal Congestion

Nasal congestion occurs when the nasal passages become blocked due to swelling in the membranes lining the nose. Those membranes are triggered by surrounding blood vessels that become inflamed due to an irritation, including a common cold or allergies. In response, the nose produces mucus to move the irritation out of the nasal passages. How you treat nasal congestion depends on the source. Congestion that is the result of seasonal allergies can be treated with oral allergy medication, much of it over-the-counter. Congestion that is the result of colds and infections can be treated with anti-congestion medications and should clear up as the infection subsides.

Saline rinses and nasal irrigation can help in the case of both colds and allergies. Pour warm, mildly salted water in one nostril, through the sinus passages and out the other nostril, taking the irritants with you. If using tap water to do nasal irrigation, boil the water first; in some parts of the country, particularly in the southeast, the water may contain small amoebas. Though ordinarily harmless, and fine when ingested, these amoebas can grow and even cause death in the nasal passages. Boiling the water eliminates this risk.

## Nosebleeds

Bleeding from the blood vessels of the nose is common, especially in children who have thinner nasal membranes. The most frequent causes of nosebleeds are dry nasal passages (due to changing seasons, climate, or certain types of heating systems), nose picking, and occasionally blunt trauma (like running into the wall).

Stopping a nosebleed is fairly straightforward. Pinch the nostrils together and compress your pinched nostrils towards your face. Lean slightly forward, wait five to ten minutes, and breathe through your mouth while waiting for the bleeding to stop. Do NOT lean backwards (which will just send the blood into your mouth, or worse, into your lungs), and keep your head above your heart (i.e., elevate the source of bleeding). Once the nosebleed stops, you can ice the nose. The average nosebleed lasts less than ten minutes. If a nosebleed goes on for longer, keeps reoccurring, or the person passes out, seek medical attention. Using a humidifier in winter and refraining from picking your nose can help prevent nose bleeds.

## Nose Fracture

A broken nose is usually the result of a blow or a fall. Symptoms generally include bruising around the nose or eyes, nasal swelling, pain and tenderness, difficulty breathing, and a crooked nose. If your nose won't stop bleeding, or your nose is markedly different in shape (very twisted), you should seek immediate medical treatment. You may have developed a septal hematoma, in which blood collects in the space between layers of the nose's cartilage, predisposing you for infections; it has to be drained. Assuming that your fracture is more straightforward, treatment generally includes resetting the bone, immobilizing it with a face mask for a few weeks, and avoiding activities that are likely to cause another break.

## Foreign Bodies in the Nose

Foreign bodies in the nose are most often placed there by children. They must be removed, because there's a chance they may be dislodged suddenly and lead to choking. While removal is best left to doctors, two techniques can be done at home.

Blow your nose. Pinch closed the nostril where the item is not located and blow out through the other nostril.

Sneeze. Sneezing provides more force than merely blowing. Again, pinch the unaffected nostril closed and sneeze out of the other one (pepper can trigger a sneeze reaction).

A third technique involves blowing a quick, but not too forceful, puff of air into the child's mouth while closing the unaffected nostril frequently works at expelling the item. The mouth and nasal passages are connected, so because the child will reflexively close off their lungs, you're in essence blowing air through the back of the nostril. However, this technique is generally recommended only under medical supervision.

Finally, sometimes the only way to remove an object is surgically.

# EARS

With an external portion made up of the pinna, that outer ridge which funnels air through the auditory canal, to the tympanic membrane, or ear drum, whose tiny bones in the middle ear send information to the cochlea, the ear is the organ that not only allows us to hear the sound of a car starting on a cloudy day, or the wind rustling through the eaves, but also to keep our balance.

## Earaches

Earaches are as they sound: pains in the ear. They occur mostly in children and have a number of possible causes, including infection, wax buildup, foreign object (including cotton swabs), and water buildup.

## Ear Infections

An ear infections is an inflammation of the ear, usually the middle ear, commonly caused by bacteria. The pain associated with ear infections is due to the fluid that builds up behind the eardrum. Children are more likely to suffer from ear infections. Most ear infections will clear up themselves without antibiotics. One study found that 97 percent of subjects' ear infections cleared within three days without antibiotics. Over-the-counter pain medications like ibuprofen and acetaminophen (aspirin can be dangerous for children) may be used to reduce pain symptoms, as can a warm or cool compress. A drop of tea tree oil in the ear canal may be beneficial for its antimicrobial effects, but it can also cause skin irritation. If the ear infection is accompanied by high fever or severe pain, antibiotics may be necessary and you should consult a doctor.

## Buildup of Wax

Although the ear naturally produces wax, too much wax can lead to a temporary loss of hearing and earaches. Use of over-the-counter peroxide-based wax removal drops can help with a buildup of wax. Alternatively, doctors can remove wax either through irrigation methods or the use of a vacuum.

## Foreign Objects in the Ear

Getting items stuck in the ear is a fairly common problem with children. There are only two circumstances and methods under which you should attempt to remove an item.

If the item is visible and the person is capable of sitting still and being cooperative, you can attempt to use blunt ended tweezers to grasp and carefully extricate the item from the ear. Don't use items like bobby pins or cotton swabs that don't have a grip. They may push the item further into the ear, potentially puncturing the eardrum.

Alternatively, you can tilt the head to the side, gently tugging the ear back and forth, which may straighten the ear canal, can dislodge the object and, in conjunction with gravity, allow it to slip out.

If the person is not cooperative, or if you can't see the object, don't try to remove it. Similarly, do not try to flush the object out. You need to see a doctor who has the tools and knowledge to remove the object.

Cotton swabs are designed for cleaning the pinnae, or external parts of the ear. They should not be use in the ear canal, because they can irritate the canal, or worse, puncture the eardrum.

## Water in the Ear

Also known as swimmers ear, this occurs when water trapped in the ear spreads a bacterial or fungal organism that causes infection. The signs and symptoms are similar to those of a severe ear infection and include fever and a feeling that your ear is blocked or full. In addition, you might have swollen lymph nodes around the ear or in the upper neck. Drainage or fluid can also leak from the ear. Treatment usually consists of using a suction device to relieve fluid in the ear, in addition to antibiotic drops. Medical care is required.

## Ruptured Eardrum

A ruptured eardrum is a hole or tear in the eardrum. Symptoms include a sudden sharp pain in the ear, or a sudden decrease in ear pain; clear, bloody, or puss-colored fluids discharged from the ear; buzzing in the ear; and partial or complete hearing loss. Confirmation of a ruptured eardrum requires a visual examination by a doctor; medical practitioners have the equipment and expertise necessary to examine the eardrum and its state. Most eardrums will heal themselves over three months. Like treating an earache, pain medication can be taken and warmth can be applied to relieve discomfort. Sometimes an eardrum requires outpatient surgery to repair it, but this is rare.

## MOUTH AND THROAT

### Sore Throats

The swollen, red, and achy feeling that accompanies a sore throat is usually the first sign of an impending cold or virus. Since the sore throat is a symptom of a larger infection, treatment is primarily focused on soothing the irritation. Pain medications and warming teas can help, as can soothing and numbing throat lozenges that contain dyclonine, benzocaine, or menthol. Occasionally sore throats are triggered by overusing the vocal cords, which leads to a scratchy feeling rather than achy one. In that case, symptoms usually abate in a day or two, but chamomile tea and refraining from talking may help.

Sometimes sore throats are caused by an infection but are not accompanied by a cold. This can be a sign of strep throat or a sexually transmitted infection (STI), especially gonorrhea.

### Strep Throat

Strep throat infections (streptococcal pharyngitis) are usually not accompanied by the traditional markers of a cold: there's no cough, sneeze, or other cold symptoms. Instead, it presents, often suddenly, as a severe throat pain, frequently accompanied by a moderate fever (over 101°F), yellow or white striations in the throat, and bright red spots on the roof of the mouth.

While most throat infections clear on their own, strep throat should be treated, usually with antibiotics, because it can turn into rheumatic fever, an infection that can cause lasting damage to the heart and even death.

## Mono

Infectious mononucleosis (or "mono") is caused by the Epstein-Barr virus. Although not everyone infected with the virus suffers symptoms, those who are symptomatic find that the virus can leave them feeling fatigued for a month or more. Teenagers and young adults aged fifteen to twenty-four are those most likely to have obvious symptoms of mono, including high to moderate fever ranging from 101°F–104°F, swollen tonsils with white patches that can be confused for strep, headache, body aches, swollen lymph nodes, and pain in the upper left part of the stomach near the spleen (it becomes enlarged in 75 percent of mono sufferers). Symptoms also include loss of appetite and, most notably, lack of energy. It can take up to two months for patients to fully recover, though the acute phase marked by fever only lasts for two weeks. Rest, hydration, and general wellness care are the prescribed course of action. It is important to resume normal activities slowly as energy levels increase. The biggest risk is to the spleen, which due to its enlarged nature can easily rupture; thus, avoid contact sports and lifting heavy objects.

## Canker Sores

Aphthous ulcers, known as canker sores, differ from cold sores in several ways: they're in the mouth, they're not contagious, and they are not caused by an infection. The exact source of their origin is unknown, though there is thought to be a genetic component. Eating diets rich in vegetables, zinc, and B12 vitamin supplements may help reduce the frequency of canker sores. Similarly, some people find that avoiding dental products, especially toothpastes that contain sodium lauryl sulfate, may help. Sodium lauryl sulfate, a lathering cleaning agent, can trigger canker sores in susceptible individuals. Treatment involves treating the mouth gently until the sore heals. Avoid consuming irritants like sour and spicy foods.

## Gum Problems

Bleeding, gum pain, and swelling can be signs of periodontal (gum) disease known as gingivitis. Gingivitis occurs when the bacteria in the mouth binds to mucus, and the particles from the food that we eat form-ing a sticky substance called plaque that binds to teeth. Over time, the bacteria in the plaque irritate the gums, which become inflamed, swell, and bleed. If gingivitis goes untreated, it can lead to periodontitis. The inflammation causes pockets along the gum line to form, the gum pulls away from the teeth, the teeth stop receiving nutrients, and tooth and bone loss follows.

Fortunately, all of this is preventable with proper dental hygiene. Brush your teeth twice a day with an American Dental Association-approved toothpaste (it will have the ADA seal on the box) for two minutes each time, floss every day, replace your toothbrush every three months, and see a dentist for general cleaning every six months. These measures will also arrest the progression of gingivitis. Once periodontitis sets in, however, more aggressive measures, including surgery, may be necessary.

## Lost Filling

Fillings are used to seal cavities, or pockets of tooth decay. They protect the tooth and its nerves from further decay. Occasionally, they fall out. When they do, you should go to the dentist and get them refilled. In the interim, you can use a temporary filling kit.

## Loose or Lost Tooth

Loose or dislodged teeth are common injuries, often the result of sports or accidents. Some tooth injuries can be prevented, especially when playing sports, by wearing a mouth guard. If a tooth is slightly loose, nothing much has to be done except resisting the childish urge to wiggle it. It should tighten up on its own over a few days. You may also want to switch to a diet consisting of mostly soft foods for two to three days to avoid making the situation worse.

If the tooth is very loose or dislodged, it needs to be reinserted within thirty minutes for the best chance at a successful reinsertion. When a tooth has been knocked out, handle it with care only by the crown; never touch the root or the portion of the tooth that connects it to the gums. Make sure that the tooth is whole and intact. If the tooth doesn't have much dirt on it, don't rinse it. If the tooth is dirty, rinse gently—do not scrub or use alcohol—to remove any dirt that may inhibit your ability to reinsert.

Have the patient rinse the mouth with warm water and reinsert the permanent tooth into the correct socket. Place a piece of gauze pad or paper over the tooth, and have the person bite down to keep it in place. You should go to the dentist or emergency room to make sure that everything is okay, and stick to a diet of soft foods for the next three days.

If the reinsertion was unsuccessful, if the tooth is in fragments, or if it's a child's baby tooth, place the tooth in small bag of whole milk, and place the bag in a cup with ice. If ice is unavailable, place the tooth in a cup of cold milk. If milk is unavailable, put the tooth in the person's mouth between their cheek and gum to prevent drying. If it's a very young child for whom choking represents a real risk, put the tooth in a cup of the person's saliva (spit). Get the tooth and the person immediately to a dentist or an emergency room.

It can hurt to have a tooth knocked out, but over-the-counter pain medication, an ice pack applied to the outside of the jaw, or sucking on a popsicle can help with symptoms.

## Digestive

The digestive system is the series of organs beginning with the mouth, stretching down to the esophagus, into the stomach, through the large intestine, into the small intestine, and out through the rectum and anus. Along with the gallbladder, pancreas, and liver, it helps you consume food and transform it into the nutrients necessary to fuel your body.

### Gas

Gas is caused by bacteria in the gut that ferment carbohydrates in the colon that weren't broken down in the small intestine. Gas can present as sharp stabbing pains in the abdomen that some confuse for heart attack. Fortunately, it is not harmful. High fiber diets, carbonated beverages, lactose intolerance, and some artificial sweeteners are all known to trigger gas. Over the counter medicines like Beano (for general gas) and lactase supplements (for lactose intolerance) can help reduce the likelihood of gas, as can dietary changes to avoid known triggers.

### Constipation

Constipation is a difficulty emptying the bowels usually associated with hardened feces. Medically, a patient is considered constipated when he or she has fewer than three bowel movements a week, and severely consti-pated with fewer than one bowel movement a week. Additional symptoms include rectal bleeding, small and hard stools, and lower abdominal dis-comfort. Most constipation is connected either to poor diets—especially diets low in fiber—or certain medications. If constipation is sudden-onset, severe, or getting worse, seek a medical professional.

Most constipation, however, can be treated by increasing fiber in the diet either through increased consumption of fruits and vegetables or consumption of fiber-based pills (usually containing psyllium husk) and beverages. Increase fiber slowly, adding a few grams of fiber every few days, because increasing fiber consumption too quickly can worsen con-stipation. Avoid taking laxatives they can make constipation worse over time. Increasing water consumption can also help to loosen your stools.

## Diarrhea

Diarrhea is the opposite of constipation; instead of stools that are too hard and heavy, stools instead are runny and watery. Symptoms of diarrhea include thin, loose, watery stool, stomach bloating, and cramps. Diarrhea has a number of different sources, including an intestinal flu, food aller-gies, diabetes, overactive thyroid, alcohol abuse, some cancers, and even spicy foods. Given that diarrhea can have so many different causes, it's important to understand when you need to call a doctor or when it's something that will resolve itself. If any of the following happens, seek medical advice: diarrhea lasts more than two days, diarrhea is accompa-nied by a fever that lasts for more than a day, you're urine is dark (a sign of dehydration), you're vomiting so severely that you can't keep down flu-ids, or you're exhibiting any of the classic signs of dehydration. Diarrhea can kill, most commonly through dehydration.

If the case of diarrhea is mild, treatment is simple. Make an effort to stay hydrated (avoid caffeine) and use hemorrhoid cream for itchiness or soreness in the rectal area from frequent bowel movements. If the diar-rhea is a particular nuisance, take an anti-diarrhea medication, but note that it doesn't stop the diarrhea. It simply acts as a chemical cork and delays its expulsion, which can be useful to continue with day-to-day life.

## Nausea

Nausea is queasiness in the stomach that often precedes vomiting. It's a sensation that can be triggered by external stimuli such as motion sickness, stress (as in panic attacks), morning sickness (in pregnant women), and illness. Illnesses that can trigger nausea include stomach viruses (symptoms include diarrhea, nausea and vomiting, fever, headache, and sore muscles), ulcers, bulimia (compulsive binge eating followed by guilty purging), food poisoning (symptoms include nausea, vomiting, runny diarrhea, stomach pain and cramping, and fever appearing one to eight hours after a meal). Most of the time nausea is harmless, but if it's persistent or accompanied by near constant vomiting that makes it difficult to rehydrate, it becomes dangerous. Treating the underlying cause will abate the symptoms.

## Severe Digestive Pain

Stomach pain, even fairly painful stomach pain, often has relatively benign origins. Constipation (from lack of fiber or dehydration), indigestion (heart burn), and gas (which occurs from the bacterial breakdown of foods such as beans, broccoli, and dairy) have frequently been mistaken at one time or another for more severe stomach ailments. Yet sometimes that pain in the stomach isn't just gas. Two possible explanations include problems with the gallbladder and appendix.

## Gallbladder

The gall bladder is a small sac below the liver that stores the bile to break down the fat that we consume. Typically, the gallbladder sits around helping us turn bacon, ice cream, and other high-fat treats into energy that we can use. If one of the ducts that transports bile from the liver gets clogged, however, we experience pain. There are two main kinds of gallbladder issues.

Biliary colic is marked by a rapid onset of pain that begins in the upper abdomen either directly under the right side of the ribs or in the center spreading to the right shoulder blade and lasting from as little as a few minutes to up to five hours. It may be accompanied by nausea and vomiting. This condition is thought to be triggered by gallstones, small cholesterol crystals that form in the gallbladder duct. Rapid weight loss, pregnancy, diabetes, and taking estrogen-based birth control are all known risk factors. Treatment is generally geared toward reducing the gallstones, and includes low-fat, fiber-rich diets, taking medication to dissolve gallstones, using sound waves to remove gallstones, and finally removing the gallbladder surgically.

Like biliary colic, acute cholecystitis occurs when gallstones block the gallbladder ducts (or more rarely as a complication of trauma known as acalculous cholecystitis). The pain experienced with acute cholecystitis is severe and lasts longer than that of biliary colic, and while it also begins in the right abdominal area and spread towards the right shoulder, moving or coughing worsens pain. The stomach will be tender to the touch, and fever, vomiting, and a feeling of the chills are all possible. Treatment is similar to biliary colic, except that infection is more likely to happen in acute cholecystitis. Since the pain lasts for so much longer, patients are more likely to suffer from dehydration and malnutrition. In clinical settings, IV drips are often used to rehydrate the patient. Cholecystitis may clear up on its own, but reoccurrence is likely; thus, surgery is common with cholecystitis.

# Appendicitis

The appendix is a thin tube just below the lower right abdomen that has no known function. One (unproven) theory is that it holds good bacteria to help repopulate the gut after diarrheal illness. The organ is perhaps best known for appendicitis, an inflammation or swelling of the appendix that forms when stool or another foreign body blocks the appendix. Roughly 7 percent of people will get appendicitis in their lifetime.

## Signs and Symptoms of Appendicitis

Classic symptoms include a loss of appetite, dull pain around the navel or upper abdomen that grows sharper as it moves downward toward the lower abdomen, stomach swelling, fever or increased temperature, and an inability to fart or otherwise release gas. Additional symptoms that can occur include painful urination and vomiting.

## Treating Appendicitis

The most common treatment for appendicitis is removal of the appendix. If the appendix becomes very inflamed, it can burst and spread the infection throughout the digestive system. However, recent studies have shown that in uncomplicated situations where the appendix is swollen but has not yet burst or perforated, appendicitis can be treated with antibiotics such as piperacillin and tazobactam, ampicillin and sulbactam, ticarcillin and clavulanate, cefepime, gentamicin, meropenem, ertapenem, and metronidazole. Of course a medical professional is best equipped to diagnose appendicitis, and antibiotics cannot be secured without a prescription.

## ORTHOPEDIC INJURIES

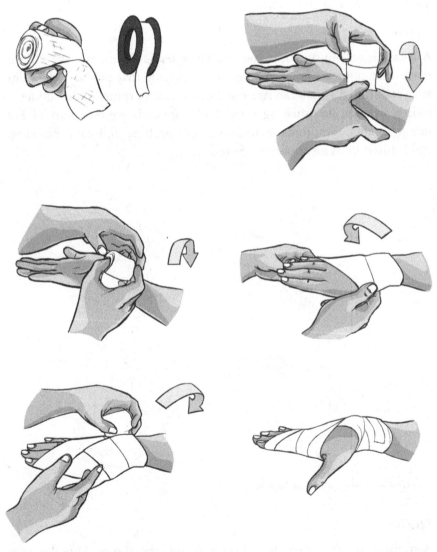

*How to bandage a hand and wrist.*

## Joint and Muscle Pain

Joint and muscle pain can be caused by a wide variety of problems ranging from typical aches and sprains to more severe injuries. Generally, joint and muscle pain comes from a source that can be easily pinpointed: muscle tension, stress, overuse, and injuring the muscle while pushing it beyond your limits. The two most common forms of joint and muscle injuries are sprains and strains.

### Sprains

A sprain is an injury where you stretch or tear a ligament—the fibrous tissue that connects bone to bone or the capsule that provides the joint with stability. A sprain can be caused by overuse or trauma, like suddenly rolling an ankle after missing a step. Ankle sprains are most common. For minor sprains, symptoms include bearable swelling and pain, bruising, and limited movement of the affected joint.

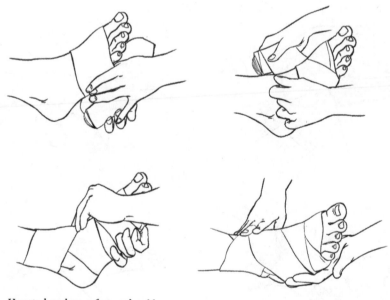

*How to bandage a foot and ankle.*

### Strains

A strain is the tearing of a muscle or a tendon, the fibrous cable that connects the muscle to the bones. They are most common in the lower back and hamstring. Symptoms include swelling, bruising, or redness, pain even at rest, pain at the affected muscle or joint, weakness of the muscle, and inability to use the muscle at all.

### Treating Sprains and Strains

Strains and sprains can generally be treated at home, but if the injury causes a popping noise or there is a significant amount of swelling, pain, fever, inability to walk, or an open wound, get emergency medical care. Treat mild sprains and strains with rest, ice, compression, and elevation. Rest the area for at least forty-eight hours. Since sprains occur most frequently in knees and ankles, braces and splints may be helpful. Ice the area for fifteen minutes at a time four to eight times a day for the first forty-eight hours. Use an elastic wrap or bandage to compress the area and elevate it higher than your heart. The use of over-the-counter pain relievers, especially ibuprofen and naproxen sodium (Aleve), may alleviate pain and reduce swelling.

In the case of muscle strains, heat pads can be used after the application of cold to soothe and relax the muscle. When applying heat or ice, never apply directly to the skin; use a cloth or a towel as a barrier.

Both the pain and swelling should begin to subside after the first few days. Reintroduce physical activities slowly, focusing on strengthening and rehabilitating the injured area. If symptoms don't improve or they get worse, see a doctor.

## Fractures and Setting Bones

A bone fracture is better known as a broken bone. While sometimes a break can be dramatic with the two parts of the bone visibly misaligned even from the outside, most fractures are tiny and difficult to diagnose even on an X-ray.

There are two kinds of fractures: open and closed. In an open fracture, the bone has penetrated the skin. Move this kind of fracture as little as possible, because movement can damage blood vessels and nerves. In addition, make sure that to control any bleeding and clean the wound before setting the bone. If there is a lot of swelling, discoloration, or numbness below the wound, there may be damage to a critical blood vessel.

Most fractures can be "set" or put into their proper place without surgery, but it is best to refrain from doing it unless there is reason to suspect it's cutting off circulation or digging into a nerve. Setting a bone without experience is risky and can damage key blood vessels. If help really is out of reach, use traction to slowly put the broken bone back into place. Only attempt this on a closed fracture.

When trying to set a bone—remember this is a last resort only when help is unavailable and won't be for some time—don't instinctively yank the bone into place. After a bone breaks, the muscles contract as a way of protecting the bone; in doing so, they make it so that bone can't ease back into place. Traction applies a consistent, firm pressure in the same plane as the bone. If it's a broken leg and the patient is lying flat on the floor, pull straight along the leg in the same direction as the bone, as though try to drag the leg along the floor. There should be no upward or downward pressure. It may be necessary to pull firmly for up to five or six minutes before the muscles release and the bone sets into place.

Once the bone sets, splint the broken bone. A splint provides the body with external support by binding it to something sturdy. As an example, for a broken finger try making a splint by placing two pens on either side of the finger, straightening the finger, and taping the whole thing together.

For something larger, like a leg, a pen clearly wouldn't do. Items like large umbrellas or wooden sticks may work. The basic rule of thumb for a splint is to stabilize the joint above and below the fracture location. For a broken lower leg, make sure that a splint immobilizes both the knee and the ankle.

## Dislocated Joints

A dislocation occurs when two bones are separated at the joint; this is most frequently caused by a blow, fall, or other sudden trauma or jolt to the joint. Symptoms include numbness or tingling at the joint (indicating damage to the nerves); pain when the patient tries to use, move, or put weight on the joint; swelling and bruising; or visible displacement. Some of the most common dislocations are the shoulder and knee.

Even if it's possible to pop the joint back into place without medical help, don't. Forcing the joint back into the socket can cause more damage than the original dislocation. Instead seek medical attention, preferably within twenty-four hours. The longer the wait, the more difficult it may become to put the joint back in the socket. A doctor's treatment will depend on the joint that has been dislocated.

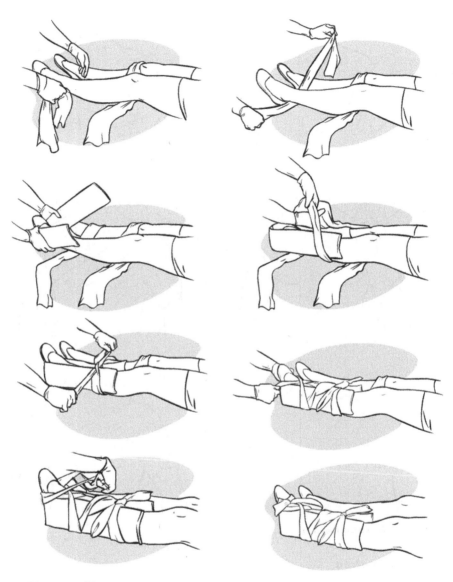

*Fashioning a splint.*

## Shoulder Dislocation

Conscious sedation, in which the body relaxes but remains conscious, is often enough for the body to pop the joint back into place. If it doesn't, the doctor will gently maneuver the shoulder bones back into place. Do not try to yank and shove the shoulder back into place because that can cause more damage.

145

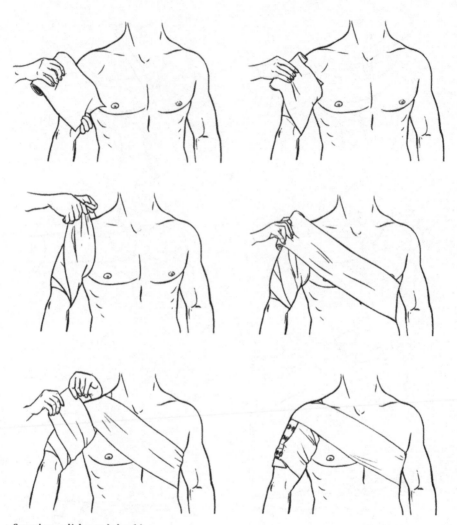

*Securing a dislocated shoulder.*

## Neck Dislocation

Immediately seek medical attention for any dislocation of the neck, since the spine and lifelong mobility are at risk. Immobilize the neck in a brace if possible. Depending on the severity of the dislocation, a doctor may prescribe surgery or a series of tension braces.

## Knee Dislocation

A doctor will likely drain the blood that's accumulated around the knee cap and gently ease it back into place. If the dislocation was the result of a minor bump or twist (with no likelihood of a break in the kneecap), it's possible to attempt to slide the kneecap back into place. If this does not work—don't force it—or if the dislocation is the result of trauma that may have broken something, splint the kneecap and get immediate medical attention. If successful, wrap the knee with an ACE bandage or other supportive tape, ice it, stay off of it as much as possible, and get to a doctor.

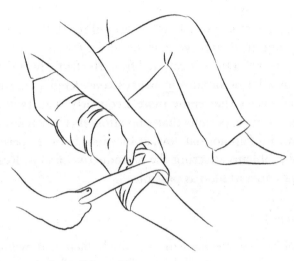

*Bandaging a dislocated knee.*

## REPRODUCTIVE

The reproductive system includes the sexual organs necessary for humans to reproduce. The systems differ in men and women, and thus reproductive care is specific to each gender.

### Menstruation

Menstruation, also known as a period, is the monthly vaginal bleeding that occurs when a woman's body sheds the inner lining of the uterus through her vagina. Most women begin menstruating between the ages of eight and fifteen (average age in the United States is twelve) and will continue menstruating for the next thirty to forty years until no longer able to reproduce, a process known as menopause.

There are several different products women use during their periods. Menstrual pads are placed on panties and collect the fluid outside of the body. Tampons are narrow columns of absorbent fabric that collect menstrual fluid from inside the vagina. Menstrual cups are soft cups usually made of medical-grade silicone shaped like a bell. Pads and tampons need to be replaced every four to eight hours depending on a woman's flow, while menstrual cups can be emptied, rinsed, and reinserted. Tampons in particular should not be kept in too long nor removed too frequently because of the risk of toxic shock syndrome (TSS); TSS causes sudden high fever and can lead to death.

A normal menstrual cycle lasts between three to five days and occurs every twenty-one to thirty-five days in adults (twenty-one to forty-five days in young teens). Day 1 is counted from the first day of the menstrual cycle. There is a lot of variance in what's considered a "normal" period, but menstrual cycles that come more frequently than twenty-one days apart, changes in flow, periods that stop altogether when a woman is not pregnant, heavier than normal flow, or bleeding between periods are possible signs of problems affecting the reproductive organs. Reach out to a health-care provider as soon as possible.

## Birth Control

Birth control is the mechanism by which men and women prevent unwanted pregnancy, usually by some form of contraceptive device.

### Diaphragm

A diaphragm is a dome-shaped (often silicone) cup inserted into the vagina, similar to a menstrual cup, where it covers the cervix. It can be placed in the vagina up to six hours before sex. For maximum efficacy, it is usually used in conjunction with spermicidal gel that should be reapplied (though the diaphragm does not need to be removed) in between sex acts.

### Hormonal Birth Control

Hormonal birth control uses various hormones, usually estrogen and progestin, to avert pregnancy by preventing ovulation. If the body doesn't ovulate, no egg is released from the ovaries, and without an egg to fertilize, a woman can't get pregnant. While hormonal birth control is used successfully by billions of women worldwide, there are some potential side effects, including mood issues, decreased libido, irregular periods,

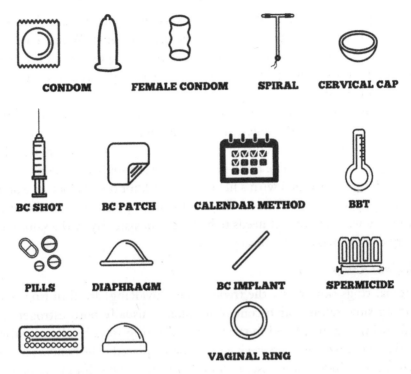

*Methods of contraception.*

heavy periods, acne (though some women experience a reduction in acne), and stroke (especially in smokers and women over the age of thirty-five). At the same time, hormonal birth control can reduce the risk of pelvic inflammatory disease, heavy periods, premenstrual syndrome (PMS), ectopic pregnancy, and ovarian cysts.

It is still possible, but rare, to get pregnant on hormonal birth control. The risk is higher when using oral contraceptives, as some women forget to take the pills on time. Additionally, many antibiotics can weaken the efficacy of hormonal birth control, so supplemental physical birth control (like condoms) should be used while taking antibiotics. Hormonal birth control needs to be prescribed by a doctor.

### Oral Contraceptives

The "Pill," also known as the birth control pill or the combination pill, uses a mixture of estrogen and progestin to prevent ovulation and thus pregnancy. Most pills mimic a twenty-eight-day ovulation cycle. Women experience menstruation-like bleeding every twenty-eight days, but since the body doesn't ovulate, this is not true menstruation. Women are able to extend periods between this false menstrual cycle by taking pills continuously and skipping the inactive "reminder pills" that are included with most packs.

There are many different formulations of the pill, each with different levels of estrogen and progestin. Different formulas work for different women, and some women discover that they need to try a few before they find a pill that works. The mini-pill is a progestin-only birth control pill. It's preferred by women with a history of or risk for blood clots, or women who experience side effects on the combination pills. Because the mini-pill is a lower dose pill, it needs to be taken consistently at the same time every day for maximum efficacy.

## Vaginal Rings

Vaginal rings (known by the trade name NuvaRing) are thin rings containing slow-release birth control hormones (usually both estrogen and progestin) that are placed in the vagina. The ring stays in place for three weeks, is removed for one week, and is then replaced. The benefits of vaginal rings include lower doses of hormones and not needing to remember to take a daily pill.

## Birth Control Implants

Birth control implants are thin, flexible pieces of plastic containing slow-release birth control hormones. Unlike vaginal rings, however, the matchstick-size strip is surgically implanted in your upper arm. It slowly releases hormones for three to five years. The upside of the implant is that you don't have to think about taking birth control for several years. However, over time many women experience a (temporary) cessation of menstruation because of the constant exposure of hormones. This goes away when the implant is removed by a doctor.

## Intrauterine Devices

Intrauterine devices, or IUDs, are T-shaped pieces of plastic placed in the uterus by medical professionals. They are most easily placed immediately after one's menstrual cycle, when the cervix is most dilated, but they can be inserted at any time provided that the patient is not pregnant. An IUD functions by interfering with sperm's ability to fertilize an egg.

They are long-term birth control devices; depending on type, they can provide up to ten years of protection. Although once only recommended for women who had previously had children, IUDs are the preferred birth control device of gynecologists for both mothers and women who have not had children. IUDs can be removed at any time, and women can become immediately pregnant after removal. The biggest risk is that an IUD can shift, rendering it ineffective; very rarely, such a shift causes a perforation the uterus, risking infection and long-term fertility. The IUD contains strings that hang down from the uterus into the upper vagina that women can check monthly to ensure that it remains properly placed.

Copper IUDs contain no hormones; rather, the structure of the device and the copper makes the uterus an inhospitable environment for sperm. Because they don't contain hormones, they are suitable for women who cannot use hormonal birth control. They provide protection for up to ten years. The most common complaints about the copper IUD include heavier menstrual flow and additional cramping. Both may subside over time as the body becomes adjusted to them.

Hormonal IUDs are generally made of plastic and contain progestin (the same hormone as in the mini-pill). They can last for three to six years. The combination of the IUD device and the hormone makes them more effective than hormones on their own. Unlike the copper IUD, women who use the hormonal IUD say that their period gets lighter over time.

### Condoms

Condoms prevent pregnancy and transmission of sexually transmitted infections (STIs) by providing a physical barrier. Generally speaking, there are two broad types of condoms: the male condom, which is designed to be placed over an erect penis before ejaculation or entering the vagina or rectum, and the female condom, which is placed in the vagina up to eight hours before sex.

Male condoms are usually made of latex, though condoms made from polyurethane (usually sold as latex-free) and sheepskin (also called natural condoms) exist for those who can't use latex condoms or would prefer the feel of other materials. It's important to note that while natural condoms protect against pregnancy, they do not protect against STI transmission. Female condoms are usually made out of polyurethane or nitrile (a synthetic rubber), so they're suitable for use by those with latex allergies.

Both female and male condoms provide protection against pregnancy. Because female condoms extend beyond the mouth of the vagina, they provide a bit more protection against STIs.

The use of oil-based lubricants should be avoided, as they can degrade both male and female condoms. You should only use water-based lubrication in conjunction with condoms.

## Reproductive Conditions
### Painful Testicle

Testicles are the small, egg-shaped organs behind the penis that produce sperm and testosterone in men. Testicles, enclosed in a sac called the scrotum, exist outside the body because sperm requires slightly cooler temperatures than the 98.6°F that is the body's normal temperature. It is common for one testicle to be smaller than the other.

There are a number of issues that can cause testicle pain—kidney stones, infection, nerve damage, hernia, enlarged veins—all of which require medical attention. One particular kind of testicle pain, testicular torsion, requires immediate medical attention to prevent permanent damage to the testicles. Testicular torsion happens when the testicle becomes twisted, cutting off blood supply to the testicle. If it goes too long without blood supply, the cells die and the testicle remains permanently damaged. It is most common among men between the ages of ten to twenty.

Pain caused by mild trauma usually doesn't require medical care. If the scrotum isn't tender to the touch, there isn't a lump, and there is no fever, pain can be treated by taking warm baths, using ice to reduce swelling, taking over-the-counter pain medications, and wearing a cup. If symptoms don't improve within a few days, seek medical care.

### Vaginal Itching and Discharge

It's important to note that some level of vaginal discharge is normal; it's how the vagina cleans itself. A small amount of white discharge at the beginning or end of the menstrual cycle, clear and watery, clear and stretchy, and even brown and bloody (during or right after the menstrual cycle) are all normal.

However, white thick discharge that has a cottage cheese–like texture may signal a yeast infection. Brown and bloody discharge outside of the menstrual cycle may be a sign of pregnancy, a miscarriage, or in very rare cases cervical cancer. Yellow and green discharge especially when accompanied by a bad smell may be a sign of a sexually transmitted vaginal infection caused by protozoa called trichomoniasis.

### Yeast Infections

Yeast infections are the result of an overgrowth of a fungus, known as candida, on the skin or mucus membranes of the vagina. Candida is always present in the vagina; yeast infections only occur when candida grow out of control due to an imbalance in the vagina. That imbalance can be triggered by diets heavy in processed sugars and grains, or by antibiotics. If it's necessary to take an antibiotic, take a probiotic or consume yogurt made with live active culture or kefir. Treatment is generally an over-the-counter medication, often creams or ointments used for one to three days. More aggressive forms of yeast infections are treated by oral medications. Because yeast infections are the result of an imbalance, the goal is to restore the balance. Boric acid capsules (made from powders, not crystals) inserted into the vagina for two weeks nightly are another treatment option. The capsules can be made at home by filling empty gelatin capsules and are considered particularly effective for treating recurrent yeast infections.

### Bacterial Vaginosis

Increased vaginal discharge accompanied by a fishy smell is a symptom of bacterial vaginosis. Like yeast infections, bacterial vaginosis results from an imbalance in the vagina. While yeast infections are fungal overgrowth, bacterial vaginosis is caused by an overgrowth in bacteria. Treatment is an oral or topical antibacterial for five to seven days. If these are totally out of reach, there's some evidence that tea tree oil and garlic ampules inserted in the vagina can help.

## Sexually Transmitted Infections

Sexually transmitted infections (STIs, also known as venereal diseases) are infections transmitted through sexual intercourse; oral, vaginal, and anal sex can transmit STIs. It is not uncommon to have an STI and yet experience no symptoms of the disease; the only way to know is through routine testing either between sexual partners or at least once a year. The only way to reduce your risk of catching an STI is to refrain from sexual activity, limit the number of sexual partners, have sex within monogamous sexual relationships with partners who have not tested positive for STIs, and/or use prophylactic contraception like condoms (which go over the genitals, reducing skin to skin contact) or dental dams (which do the same for the mouth for oral sex).

## Gonorrhea

Gonorrhea is a bacterial infection sometimes called "the clap" or "the drip." Gonorrhea is not limited to growing in the genital regions, it can also grow in the mouth, throat, and anus. Some men and most women with gonorrhea never show symptoms of the disease. When symptoms do present, in men they generally appears as painful or swollen testicles, a white, yellow, or green discharge, or a burning sensation when urinating. Women also experience a painful or burning sensation when urinating, as well as increased vaginal discharge and vaginal bleeding in between menstrual cycles. Antibiotic pills are the most common treatment.

## Hepatitis B

Hepatitis B is a virus that causes inflammation of the liver. It is most commonly, though not exclusively, spread by intimate sexual contact. Symptoms of hepatitis B infection include abdominal pain, nausea, vomiting, dark urine, fever, yellowish skin, joint pain, weakness, and fatigue. While hepatitis B may clear up on its own, chronic cases require a lifetime of treatment and may lead to liver cirrhosis or liver cancer. There is no cure yet, though a cancer treatment in clinical trials looks promising. Hepatitis B can be prevented with a vaccine given over the course of three to four shots.

## Herpes

Herpes is an infection caused by one of two viruses: herpes simplex virus types 1 (HSV-1) and 2 (HSV-2). Herpes simplex 1 usually, but not always, presents as cold sores or fever blisters in the mouth, while herpes simplex 2 usually presents as genital blisters or ulcers. (It is also possible to get an HSV-1 infection on your genitals.) The small blisters will often leak a clear fluid, scab over, and heal in up to two weeks. Many people infected with the herpes virus never present symptoms because their immune systems suppress it. Others may have reoccurring outbreaks (varying in frequency) characterized by the emergence of the herpes sores.

There's no cure for herpes, though some treatments to suppress outbreaks do exist. For women who are pregnant or thinking about becoming pregnant, it is important to note that the disease can increase the risk of miscarriage and can be transmitted to the baby; neonatal herpes is a potentially life-threatening illness. Getting tested or telling a doctor about a herpes infection can allow for preventive measures that increase the likelihood of a child's survival and reduce the risk of passing on the disease.

When the herpes virus is symptomatic, the sores shed active viruses. Refrain from touching them or the fluids that emerge from them because it is possible to transfer the virus to other people or to other parts of the body, like the eyes. Because herpes sores are open wounds, they increase the risk of not only transmitting herpes to others, but also of catching other STIs, especially HIV (particularly with genital herpes). It is best to refrain from intimate contact during an outbreak.

### Human Papillomavirus

Human papillomavirus (HPV), a group of one hundred fifty related viruses, is the most common sexually transmitted infection in the United States. In many cases the virus goes away on its own, but when it doesn't, it can trigger genital warts and even cancer. A vaccine for some strains of HPV exists, and the CDC recommends that all boys and girls aged eleven to twelve years old should get vaccinated. If they were not vaccinated when younger, there are catch-up vaccines for men through the age of twenty-one and women through the age of twenty-six.

### HIV/AIDS

Human immunodeficiency virus (HIV) attacks and weakens the immune system and leaves it less capable of fighting off disease and infections. When first infected with HIV, symptoms include a slight fever, sore throat, or rash. Most people with HIV show no symptoms of the disease, sometimes for as long as ten years. At some point (sooner than later if you go without treatment), HIV will weaken the immune system to the point that the body can no longer fight off infections. This stage is called acquired immunodeficiency syndrome (AIDS).

There is no cure for the disease, though antiretroviral therapy treatments can slow the progression of the virus (especially in early stages) allowing people to live long, healthy, fruitful lives. The sooner treatment begins after infection, the better the long-term prognosis. Post-exposure prophylaxis (PEP) medications should be taken in the first seventy-two hours after possible exposure to prevent infection (although success is less than 100 percent).

### Syphilis

Syphilis is a bacterial disease that in early stages causes a painless but infectious sore on the genitals or in the mouth. Secondary symptoms include a rash, flu-like symptoms, and hair loss. The disease can easily be treated with a shot of penicillin. If left untreated, however, the disease can cause permanent brain damage and even death. Syphilis is particularly risky for pregnant women, because it can lead to complications in childbirth including low birth weight, premature birth, and even stillbirth.

### Trichomoniasis

Trichomoniasis is an infection of the vagina caused by protozoa, and a common symptom is yellow and green discharge, sometimes accompanied by a bad smell. Trichomoniasis is usually treated by a course of antibiotics called metronidazole. Left untreated, it can be passed onto others and cause low birth weight babies. Babies with a low birth weight are more likely to suffer from a number of health issues.

Trichomoniasis can be prevented by only having sex with one partner who you know to be uninfected and who also only has sex with you (monogamy) as well as using condoms when having sex.

## OTHER COMMON AILMENTS

## Common Cold

It begins with a tickle or a sneeze. Within a day or so, it turns into the dreaded cold with sneezing, sore throat, runny nose, congestion, and even fever. Recovery can take up to fourteen days, and there's no cure. The common cold is a viral infection of the upper respiratory system. Because colds are caused by viruses, antibiotics aren't effective. What does work is drinking lots of fluids, getting plenty of rest, and not forgetting the chicken soup; the old wives' tale around chicken soup's medicinal value is increasingly supported by a number of scientific studies. Lozenges, tea (especially chamomile), and cough drops can help sooth an irritated throat. Over-the-counter cold medications can be effective in treating symptoms, but be careful. Although symptoms may go away, the infection can last longer than most people expect, and they are still sick and possibly infectious. And, as always, the best solution is prevention. Wash hands frequently, sneeze into the elbow (and teach others to do the same), and get plenty of rest. Lack of sleep makes us particularly prone to catching colds. If symptoms don't improve after a few days, or if symptoms get worse (high fever and wracking chills), it may not be a cold at all, but rather the flu.

## Flu

While the common cold can be caused by over a hundred different subsets of two viruses, (adenovirus or coronavirus), the flu is caused by just one: the influenza virus. Unlike the cold, most strains of the flu can be prevented by a vaccine. Vaccination is very important, because while most people easily recover from the common cold, the flu can be deadly. Symptoms of the flu include a fever (as high as 104°F), aching joints, and infection in the lungs, not uncommonly leading to pneumonia. Flu patients can sound like there's rattling in the chest when they breathe. In children it, often infects the intestinal tract causing diarrhea and vomiting.

Treatment for the flu is similar to a cold: get plenty of rest and use over-the-counter medications to deal with symptoms. However, don't take medications that will stop productive coughs. Nasal irrigation with saline (salt water solution) can clear respiratory pathways and help flush out the virus. Avoid being around others until twenty-four hours after the fever dissipates to avoiding infecting others. If the flu lasts longer than seven to ten days or if symptoms worsen, seek medical attention. With the flu in particular, an ounce of prevention is worth a pound of cure. Get vaccinated every year, and follow good hygiene: hand washing, avoiding shared cups and utensils, covering coughs and sneezes, and getting plenty of rest.

Particularly if the flu-sufferer is young, elderly, or immunocompromised, it is imperative to seek medical attention if possible. In the United States alone, over thirty-six thousand people die from complications of the flu each year, and two hundred thousand are hospitalized. It is possible to spread the flu even if asymptomatic, so if exposed, be careful to visit a doctor and avoid contact with those with weaker immune systems who are more susceptible to contracting the flu and have not received the vaccine. Getting a flu shot each year will not only prevent development of the flu, but will protect others, especially those who cannot get flu shots, from getting sick. These people include children younger than six months, the elderly, people with allergies to eggs and other ingredients in the vaccine, and people suffering from illnesses that compromise their immune system, like Guillain-Barré syndrome (GBS).

## Fevers

Fevers are a temporary increase in body temperature. A fever isn't an illness itself, and it rarely comes alone; other symptoms can help diagnose the underlying illness, which can be caused by viruses, bacteria, fungi, drugs, and toxins. Body temperature is measured using a thermometer—oral, rectal, under-arm (axillary), in-ear, or forehead depending on the model. Low-grade fevers are generally between 100°F–102°F in adults, but for infants (zero to six months), seek immediate medical care. Any temperature above 103°F is considered a high-grade fever, and can indicate a serious illness (and could even lead death); seek immediate medical attention.

It's important to note that fever is actually one way that the body fights off infections; elevated temperatures make some immune cells work better. While fever can be uncomfortable, reducing it shouldn't necessarily be the first course of action, especially if the fever is low to moderate. If a high-grade fever is not responding to fever-reducing medications—ibuprofen, aspirin, or acetaminophen—seek medical attention.

IMPORTANT: Aspirin should never be given to anyone under the age of eighteen due to the risk of Reye's syndrome, a rare but serious condition that causes the brain to swell.

## Hemorrhoids

Hemorrhoids are swollen veins in the anal canal that, though painful, are rarely serious. They're often triggered due to straining actions as a result of diarrhea and constipation, pregnancy that puts increased pressure on pelvic blood vessels, or the pressure of being overweight. Symptoms include rectal pain, bleeding during bowel movements, and itching. Hemorrhoids can be internal, within the walls of the rectal canal, or external, where they show up as a lump under the skin. Since rectal bleeding in particular can be a sign of anal cancer, it is best to get a diagnosis confirmed by a physician. Treatment may include slowly increasing fiber in the diet and using over-the-counter anti-itch ointments and stool softeners to help alleviate symptoms and allow the area to heal. Limit the amount of time spent sitting. Hemorrhoid cushions, small pillows with a cut out in the center, may ease pressure on the area. If symptoms are severe, surgical procedures, including the use of a laser to burn away hemorrhoidal tissue, may be necessary.

## Hernia

A hernia occurs when an organ moves from the cavity where it normally rests and bulges through weak muscle. There are several types of hernia, including those of the abdomen, femoral artery, umbilical area, stomach, diaphragm, and incision site. More than 75 percent of hernias are abdominal wall hernias. They most frequently occur in men and are usually caused by increased pressures in the area, such as lifting weights that are too heavy, straining during bowel movements, gaining too much weight in the stomach, muscle strain due to chronic cough, or dialysis associated with treating kidney failure. Abdominal wall hernias can be indirect, following the path made by the testicles while a man developing as a fetus in the womb. This kind of hernia can happen at any age and generally presents as a bulge in the groin. A direct hernia happens when it protrudes on the side of the abdomen wall. Direct hernias are most common in middle age, because as we get older our abdominal muscles get weaker. Hernias require surgical repair.

Some ways of preventing hernias include lifting heavy objects with the knees and not the back, avoiding lifting weights that are too heavy, avoiding straining during bowel movements, maintaining a healthy weight, treating severe coughs, and not smoking (which can cause chronic coughing).

## PSYCHOLOGICAL CARE

While much of our focus is often spent improving our physical wellbeing—typically through diet and exercise—psychological care of our mental and emotional wellbeing is equally as important. An increasing number of studies show that there's a strong mind-body connection; regular exercise can help stave off mild to moderate depression, while depression has been linked to a host of health problems, such as heart disease. Other studies have shown that psychological stress can slow healing of wounds and cuts by as much as 25 percent. Taking care of your mental hygiene, should be as much a part of your daily regimen as brushing your teeth, and taking a bath.

There are several techniques to improve psychological wellbeing. First, be aware of how the mind reacts to failure; it can trick a person into stopping too soon and reinforce negative beliefs. Negative attitudes about failure often emerge from a fixed mindset: "If I didn't succeed this time, I'll never succeed." Instead, recognize that failures are feedback mechanisms that encourage improvement and make success sweeter. Crossing the line finish line of a marathon, writing a book, or building a home might not bring a sense of accomplishment if they weren't also *hard*, challenging the limits of our abilities, making us deal with setbacks, and trying our patience.

## Don't Be Your Own Worst Enemy

The mental voice we use to speak about ourselves is often incredibly self-critical. It repeats on a near constant basis all of our supposed flaws, foibles, stumbles, and falls. And worse, it frequently does so when we're hurting from the sting of a recent rejection. When turned down for a job offer, we don't merely recoil from the sting of this rejection; our mind will mentally catalog every job rejection, and then move onto every other rejection we've ever experienced, down to that time we weren't chosen for a dodgeball team in kindergarten. This form of overthinking, known as rumination, is emotionally harmful. If hit by the urge to ruminate, think of something else, anything else. Studies show that just a few minutes of distraction from our rumination can improve mental health and wellbeing in just a few days. Does this mean that we should never critically analyze aspects of our lives? No. But assess, and move on. Don't spend hours, days, weeks of your life rehashing a mistake made in a business meeting or the million-dollar lottery ticket accidentally flushed down the toilet.

## Practice Gratitude

We often spend so much time focused on what we don't have and mired in envy. Focusing on what we DO have reduces feelings of jealousy, resentment, and regret. At the same time, it enhances empathy, reduces aggression, improves relationships with other people, and even helps us sleep better. To practice gratitude, just scribble down a list of things to feel grateful for once a week in a journal. And, when good things happen, feel good about them.

## Stress Management

When it comes to stress of either the body and mind, like the fairytale of Goldilocks and the three bears, are seeking the right level: not too much or too little, but just right. Stress is what kicks in when we see that afore-mentioned bear, what creates a much-needed tunnel vision right before we go on stage to speak publicly before a crowd of hundreds. Stress can feel exhilarating; it's why we ride rollercoasters and hurl ourselves out of airplanes. On the other hand, *sustained* stress, the stress of dealing with an unhappy work environment for months or years, juggling multiple jobs without much sleep, or the insecurity that comes with unhealthy living environments, can make us sick, literally. In the short term, we might find ourselves sleeping or eating too much to compensate. Over the long term, however, we can end up with heart disease, muscle tension, unclear thinking, and vulnerability to colds and other infections. The question, then, is how do we manage stress?

First, make a conscious decision as to how much stress you choose to add to your life. You can say no to tasks that add more stress than pleasure to your life. You don't have to or need to do everything. You don't have to work so hard to deal with the stress in your life if the level of stress in your life is manageable.

We can't always manage the stress is in our lives. A family member might fall ill and we become their personal caretaker, or employment changes at work can leave us handling more work but without any extra time. We can, however, manage our response to these increasing levels of stress. As little as twenty minutes of meditation, especially mind-fulness meditation, a day can help our mind and body's better manage stress. Mindfulness meditation works by encouraging us to focus our attention fully on the present moment. This might begin with exercises that focus on the breath, or taking a walk through our neighborhood while focusing on how our foot strikes the ground, or the tension in our gait.

Additional suggestions include properly managing your time, so that you can avoid the stressful scramble that comes with trying to complete tasks at the last minute. Eat well and exercise regularly, so that not just that your body, but also your brain has what it needs to best regulate your moods. Make time for friends, family, and other loved ones, because loneliness kills. By some estimates, chronic loneliness increases likelihood of death by 14 percent. It also increases cholesterol, blood pressure, and the risk of depression. Finally, make time for hobbies and activities that you enjoy.

## Anxiety and Panic Attacks

Anxiety is a persistent, excessive sense of worry about everyday things. Although anxiety and fear both trigger similar physical responses, including racing heartbeat, they are different. Fear might manifest as a natural reaction to stumbling across a bear in the woods. Anxiety is still worrying about that bear six months later from your home in the middle of Los Angeles. If you routinely expect the worst, find yourself anxious without a reason, and anticipate disaster—financial, environmental, or familial—at every turn, you might be suffering from general anxiety disorder. If so, you're not alone; roughly 3.6 million Americans have general anxiety disorder, though you should check with a mental health practitioner for official diagnosis.

Sometimes, that persistent feeling of anxiety comes with panic attacks, the sudden onset of an intense feeling of fear or discomfort that is not related to your immediate surroundings. They can include sweating, a pounding heart, nausea or abdominal distress, vomiting, feeling dizzy, chest pain, shortness of breath, a feeling that you're "going crazy," numbness and tingling sensations, or a fear of dying.

Dealing with general anxiety and panic attacks depends on the frequency and severity of the symptoms. If they're interfering with daily life—causing you to procrastinate on work or avoid everyday situations like going to the supermarket or to school to avoid the symptoms—you should absolutely consult a mental health practitioner. If your symptoms are occasional and more a nuisance, try these tips to see if they help before seeking medical attention.

## Tips for Dealing with Panic and Anxiety Attacks

1. Acknowledge that you're having a panic attack/feeling anxious. Panic and anxiety feeds on itself; if you start panicking that you're panicking, you are only going to make the situation worse. Similarly, there is nothing more annoying than feeling anxious and then feeling anxious about feeling anxious.

2. In the midst of a panic attack, tell the attack to bring its worst. While this may sound paradoxical, challenging your attack may help ease symptoms by helping you to recognize that the attack is reacting to situations that are not harmful to you, or, if the situation is stressful, is impeding your ability to deal with the situation effectively.

3. Distract, distract, distract. Anxious about a report that you have to turn in? Don't think about it, think about something else, or think about how you're coping with your panic and anxiety. Tell yourself that "you've got this" or ask yourself what your favorite superhero would do in your situation. The less you identify your sense of self with the sense of panic—while acknowledging that the panic or anxiety exists—the better off you'll be.

4. Expose yourself to the source of your panic or anxiety. The more you avoid it, the more it has a grip on you. This doesn't mean you have to overcome your anxiety of deep water by jumping into the deep end of the pool; you can ease in from the shallow side.

# Depression

Depression is a very common mood disorder marked by intense, long-lasting periods of sadness. While we all feel sad sometimes, depression does not have causal factors; if there are causal factors, the depressed person is unable to adapt. It's normal to feel incredibly sad after the loss of a parent, for example. But you should, on balance, feel better three months after their loss than you did immediately after it happened. It takes a while to recover from serious loss or trauma, but the general trajectory of recovery is positive.

With depression, however, you remain persistently sad or your symptoms get worse. Activities that you once enjoyed become less appealing. You may be plagued by a sense of worthlessness and a lack of hope, both for your present condition and the future. You may even think you and the world would be better off without you.

Physically, you may feel tired, you may have trouble sleeping or sleep too much, your body may ache for no reason, and you may eat too much or too little. You may self-medicate with drugs or alcohol. You have a difficult time getting through the day and may call out sick from work a lot. Your friends may start to complain that they haven't seen you or heard from you in a while. If these symptoms are familiar, seek get medical help. Depression is treatable with counseling and prescription medication.

## Treating Mild to Moderate Depression

Treatment for depression depends on the severity. Here are some tips for dealing with mild to moderate depression. For moderate to severe depression, seek medical advice.

Regular exercise not only boosts endorphins in the short term, but over the long term it encourages the brain to rewire itself in small ways. The best exercise for depression is the exercise you most enjoy and can easily stick with. Depression makes you less resilient to setbacks, so throwing hurdles of perfection is the disease talking not you. If you like running, run; if you like bicycling, bike; if you like dancing, dance. If you've been feeling socially isolated, exercise is an opportunity to socialize more, perhaps by joining a group activity. Martial arts in particular are a sport that are both individualized and group-centric in nature. If you pick an exercise you don't like, don't stick with it just for the sake of sticking with it. Try a few before you commit.

Set a routine and stick to it. Your routine should not be jam-packed, since it's less about what you do then just doing it. The goal is to integrate beneficial activities into your life while minimizing unhealthy activities like excessive television watching, alcohol consumption, and oversleeping.

Set goals. Depression can make you feel as though you're incapable of accomplishing anything. Set small goals that prove depression is a liar; it can even be as small as washing the dishes or arriving on time at work. Success builds on success. As you feel better, you can add more challenging goals until you're back to healthy activity levels.

Eat healthfully. Food has a tremendous impact on mood. Try to eat lots of vegetables and fruits. Stick with complex grains and reduce alcohol consumption.

Get enough sleep. Depression can cause people to either not sleep enough or to sleep too much. Your goal is to get enough, which for most people is seven to nine hours a night.

Don't be so serious. Make an effort to have fun and do healthy activities that you enjoy, be it hanging with friends, doing something musical or artistic, or taking a moment to enjoy your surroundings.

If these don't work, or if you find your symptoms getting worse, especially including suicidal thoughts, reach out to a mental health practitioner for help. There are a host of options available to you including psychotherapy, cognitive behavioral therapy, and prescription medicines that can help ease your symptoms.

**Suicidal Thoughts** are thoughts about how to kill oneself. They can range from fleeting thoughts to detailed plans. If you're experiencing suicidal thoughts, seek help immediately. You don't deserve to think that life is not worth living. You can reach out to your psychiatric counselor or call the U.S. National Suicide Prevention Lifeline at 1-800-273-8255.

### Postpartum Depression

This is depression that sets in after giving birth to a child. Some amount of the "baby blues"—crying, feeling overwhelmed, mood swings, and irritability after giving birth—is normal. The body is readjusting its hormone levels post-pregnancy, and the result can be emotional turmoil. The baby blues generally begin shortly after birth (a day or two) and subsides within one to two weeks. Postpartum depression, however, mimics the symptoms of depression and can begin as long as six months after birth. In addition to symptoms common to depression, women suffering from postpartum depression will find that they have difficulty bonding with their child. It's important to recognize that postpartum depression is serious, but it is treatable. Seek medical advice.

### Seasonal Affective Disorder

Seasonal affective disorder (SAD), also called seasonal depression, is depression triggered by the seasons. While many people suffer from SAD in winter due to decreased sunlight, some people suffer from SAD in spring and summer as well. Fall/winter SAD is marked by moodiness, cravings for foods like carbohydrates, a heavy feeling, and a tendency to oversleep. It's generally treated with light therapy via exposure to specific sources of light that safely mimic the sun. Medications and counseling can also be helpful.

# CHAPTER 7

## FULL-ON MEDICAL EMERGENCIES

### RECOGNIZING AND TREATING LIFE-OR-DEATH INJURIES AND COPING WITH SEVERE PAIN

## SHOCK

Shock happens when there isn't enough blood flowing through the body. It's commonly the result of serious injuries like those from car accidents, but can stem from other sources. There are five kinds of shock.

- ☐ **Septic** shock comes from an underlying infection within the body
- ☐ **Anaphylactic** shock comes from an allergic reaction
- ☐ **Cardiogenic** shock is usually caused by an underlying heart condition
- ☐ **Hypovolemic** shock comes from a loss of blood (either from an external injury or an internal injury in which the bleeding is not immediately visible)
- ☐ **Neurogenic** shock comes from damage to the spinal cord

### Symptoms of Shock

Symptoms of shock include cold and clammy skin that may appear grayish depending on the person's skin tone, low blood pressure, enlarged pupils, inability to urinate, bluish tint to the lips and fingernails, and heavy sweating. If the person is conscious, they will cycle through a number of varying emotional states including confusion, disorientation, anxiousness, and agitation. They may feel dizzy or faint, and complain of feeling tired or chest pain, feel nauseous or even vomit.

### Treating Shock

When a person displays symptoms of shock, immediately call for emergency services. Shock is a serious condition, and it needs expertise to properly diagnose and treat. Then begin a process of checking the person's

ABCs: airways, breathing, and circulation (see more on pages 111-112). Check to make sure that their airway is unblocked and that they're breathing. If possible, check and monitor their blood pressure to make sure that it isn't declining further.

If the patient is not breathing, begin CPR. If person is breathing, is conscious, and doesn't have any injuries to the head, neck, spine, or legs, put them in the shock position. The shock position is flat on the back with legs elevated more than twelve inches. Do not move the person, unless keeping them in that location will further endanger their lives. Do not let them eat or drink anything, because it's common for them to choke if they pass out while eating. Provide basic first aid to any visible injuries, including dressing (with clean materials if possible) and applying pressure to bleeding wounds. You also want to keep the person as warm as possible; use jackets, blankets, towels, and even plastic bags to help the person stay warm. If the person vomits or is bleeding from the mouth and does not have a spinal injury, turn the body over to the side to prevent choking. You should also use your fingertips to clear any vomit from the person's mouth so he or she doesn't choke on it.

Septic shock is treated with large amounts of fluid to tackle the patient's dehydration along with antibiotics to tackle the infection. For anaphylactic shock, epinephrine and steroids are used. Cardiogenic shock frequently requires surgery to remove the blockage, while hypovolemic shock is treated intravenously with saline in mild cases, but in severe cases blood transfusions are necessary. Finally, because damage to the spinal cord is often both irreversible and has repercussions that occur throughout the body, neurogenic shock is the most difficult shock to treat. Immobilization, fluids, and anti-inflammatory medications are the most frequent course of action. The difficulties in identifying and treating the varying forms of shock are why it's so critical to reach out to a medical expert.

# BREATHING DIFFICULTY
## Checking Vitals

When someone is having difficulty breathing, it is important to check his or her vital signs to attempt to identify the source of the problem. Vital signs include temperature, pulse rate, respiration rate, and blood pressure; these are useful in monitoring or identifying a medical problem.

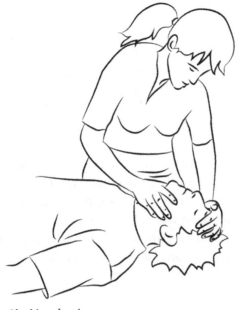

*Checking the airway.*

### Temperature

A body's temperature should generally hover around 98.6°F, though normal temperatures can be as low as 97.8°F and as high as 99°F for a healthy adult depending on time of day, food and fluid consumption, and activity level. If a person has just run a marathon on a warm day, a higher body temperature can be normal.

Temperature is measured using a thermometer. Methods of taking a temperature include oral (under the tongue), rectal (in the rectum), axillary (under the arm/in the armpit), tympanic (by ear), and temporal artery (skin of forehead). Temperatures taken rectally are 0.5°F–0.7°F higher than those taken my mouth, while temperatures taken using the axillary method are 0.3°F–0.4°F cooler than those taken by mouth. Purchase a thermometer type for your preferred form of taking temperatures. Most temperatures today are measured using digital thermometers, because they're accurate, easy to read, and quick. Traditional glass thermometers are slower and prone to breakage; until recently, they contained mercury, a neurotoxin that is hard to clean up properly in the case of breakage. Now there are a number of glass, non-mercury thermometers on the market.

## Pulse Rate

The pulse rate is the measure of the heart rate, or how many time per minute a heart beats, as well as the strength of the pulse. A normal pulse rate is between 60 and 100 beats per minute (bpm), though it can be higher if you've just hopped off of the treadmill and lower, near 40 bpm, if you're an athlete who does a lot of cardiovascular exercise like running.

To measure a pulse, press the first and second fingertips on the arteries pressing against either the inside of the elbow (where blood frequently gets drawn during medical examinations), the inside of the wrist, or the side of the neck (where the jaw meets the neck, making sure to press lightly and only press on one side of the neck so as not to block blood flow to the brain). Using a stopwatch or a clock, count the pulse for sixty seconds (or for twenty seconds and then multiply for by three) to get the number of beats per minute.

## Respiration Rate

The respiration rate is the number of breaths a person takes per minute. The easiest way of measuring respiration rate, especially in another person, is to watch how many times their chest rises in a minute. Normal respiration rate for an adult at rest is twelve to sixteen breaths per minute.

## Blood Pressure

Blood pressure is the force of blood pushing against the artery walls. When blood pressure is low, the brain and extremities may not be getting enough blood; this could lead to fainting or simply feeling cold. If blood pressure is high, patients are more likely to suffer from cardiovascular diseases like stroke or heart attack. Normal blood pressure for an adult is less than 120 mm HG systolic pressure (the upper number) and less than 80 mm HG (the lower number). Blood pressure is too low if it drops suddenly or if it starts to cause symptoms. The only way to check blood pressure is with a medical device.

# Choking

Choking happens when an object blocks the flow of air through the windpipe. This most commonly happens with food, because the esophagus (for food) and the larynx (for air) share a tube before branching off. If the windpipe was directly connected to the sinuses, it would be possible to breathe and eat at the same time. This unique structure is what enables us to speak, but also to choke; occasionally food goes down the wrong branch into our windpipe instead of our food pipe. Choking is a defensive mechanism to keep food out of our lungs, which could cause an infection.

How can you tell if a person is choking? In an adult, someone might suddenly be unable to talk, coughing, gagging, signaling with hands, clutching the throat (a pretty universal sign of choking), wheezing, passing out, or turning blue (the last two signs are rather serious). In infants, the signs are subtler: difficulty breathing, a weak cry, and/or a weak cough.

If a person is choking, but coughing and able to communicate on some level, don't intervene—they have a partial airway obstruction that will likely resolve itself. Don't offer water either, because liquids may fill the gap that turns a partial airway obstruction into a complete airway obstruction. If the person is not communicating or the coughing has stopped, you can try what the American Heart Association calls abdominal thrusts.

### Abdominal Thrusts for Choking Victims

Standing behind the person, lean them slightly forward as if the victim were a rag doll that can't stand completely upright. Turn one hand into a fist, wrap arms around the victim and grab the fist in the open hand, and rest the arms on the person's stomach right above their rib cage, and make a quick hard movement both inward and upward. This movement may assist the person in coughing up the stuck object. Repeat until the obstruction clears or the person loses consciousness. If the person loses consciousness, perform CPR (see pages 172-173).

In infants under the age of one, abdominal thrusts won't work. Instead pick the child up and angle them so that the head is tilted downward but still supported; hit them on the back with five firm blows, followed by five chest thrusts using the pads of two or three fingers in the center of the infant's chest to compress the breast bone five times about one and a half inches. Repeat until the obstruction is clear. If the child turns blue or loses consciousness, perform CPR (see pages 172-173).

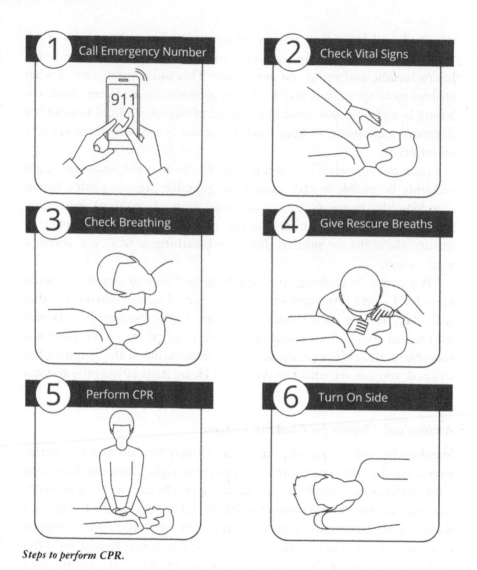

*Steps to perform CPR.*

## CPR

CPR stands for cardio pulmonary resuscitation. Performing CPR tries to resuscitate the patient, or keep a person alive until assistance can come, by mimicking the movements of the heart and lungs.

## Performing CPR

- Open airway by tilting the head, lifting the chin, and clearing away with your hands any obvious obstructions.
- Check for breathing for no more than ten seconds. Occasional gasps are not breathing.
- For an adult or child, put the heel of your hand in the center of the chest at the nipple line. For an infant, use two fingers on the breastbone.
- Press down two inches for an adult or child, making sure not to press down on the ribs; press down an inch and a half on an infant, making sure not to press down at the end of the breast bone.
- You're going to do thirty chest compressions at the rate of one hundred compressions a minute (roughly equal to the beat of the Bee Gees' "Stayin' Alive" or Queen's "Another One Bites the Dust"). Check to see if the person is breathing.
- If the patient is not breathing, you should pinch the nose to create a tight seal, breathe two puffs of air into the mouth (rescue breaths), and repeat the chest compressions. Repeat until the person starts breathing or help arrives.

People have recovered successfully from as much as thirty minutes of CPR, so it is important to continue chest compressions and rescue breaths until help arrives or you become too exhausted to continue.

For children and infants, give five rescue breaths, blowing more gently, instead of two. Do a round of CPR before calling for assistance, and in the case of a baby, cover both the infant's mouth and nose with your mouth. Chest compressions should also be done with less force.

## Asthma Attacks

Asthma is a condition in which a person's airways periodically become inflamed, a period known as an asthma attack. The airways become narrower and produce extra mucus, making it harder to breathe. Many sufferers

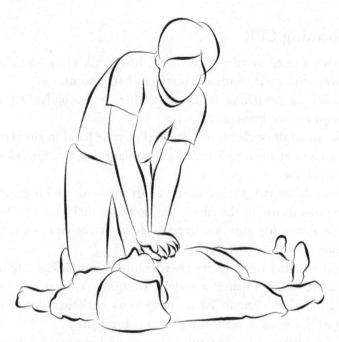

*Performing chest compressions. Try singing the song "Stayin' Alive" to help maintain the correct interval.*

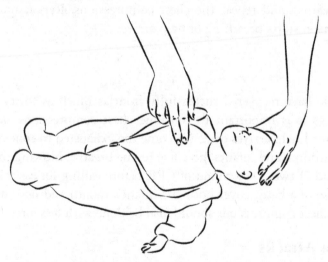

**Perform less forceful chest compressions on an infant or young child.**

describe trying to breathe during an asthma attack as similar to trying to breathe through a straw. The symptoms of an asthma attack include wheezing, shortness of breath, and coughing.

Asthma has a number of known triggers, or asthmagens. These include cold weather (cover nose and mouth with a scarf before venturing outdoors), hot humid weather with poor air quality, mold, and the presence of vermin, like mice and roaches, in a home. In addition, allergies such as to dust and pets, can also trigger an attack. Avoid these asthmagens when possible.

### Responding to an Asthma Attack

Asthma patients should work with medical professionals to prescribe a course of treatment that both minimizes the likelihood of an attack and provides the necessary medications should an attack arise. Asthma is treated through a mix of long-term maintenance medications, which are slower acting but help to reduce the inflammation that many asthma sufferers have, even between attacks. They help decrease the likelihood of an attack and should be taken regardless of whether or not a person appears symptomatic.

Quick-relief medications, also called rescue inhalers, are typically inhaled directly into the lungs where they open up airways and relieve the symptoms of an asthma attack, frequently within minutes. These drugs don't have a lasting effect, however, and should be used in conjunction with maintenance medications.

### What to Do If You Don't Have Access to Medication

If, for some reason, someone has an asthma attack and is caught without appropriate medicines, there are steps to take to survive the attack. First, move away from any possible triggers. Second, use the Buteyko breathing method developed by Russian doctor Konstantin Buteyko to prevent hyperventilation.

Hyperventilating makes asthma worse by lowering carbon dioxide levels in the blood so that airways constrict further to conserve it. Instead of breathing deeply, take a small breath in, a small breath out, and a holding breath before returning to a normal breath. The method is actually quite detailed, so exploring it before it is needed is strongly encouraged; there are training classes and a training materials online.

Finally, drink caffeine. Hot caffeinated drinks like coffee or tea relax airways and decrease the lungs' response to irritants. This may provide at least some temporary release. It can take a few hours for the caffeine to kick in, however.

## Pneumonia

Like asthma, pneumonia is an inflammation of the lungs. In a pneumonia patient, the alveoli, or air sacs of the lungs, become inflamed as a result of an infection. At its worst, the lungs can fill with fluid or puss.

### Diagnosing and Treating Pneumonia

Pneumonia is characterized by fever (which may be less common in older adults), shaking "teeth chattering" chills, fast, shallow breathing, and a feeling of constantly being short of breath, having fast heartbeat, and experiencing chest pain that is made worse by coughing or merely breathing in.

Pneumonia can be caused by bacteria, viruses, fungi, or other sources. It is difficult to identify the source, and doctors may use physical exams, X-ray images, blood tests, and cultures in making diagnoses. Nonbacterial pneumonia is often more gradual and less severe. People frequently don't even realize that they have non-bacterial pneumonia. Bacterial pneumonia is usually treated with antibiotics and proper home care, which includes drinking plenty of fluids to prevent dehydration and taking fever reducers such as acetaminophen (aspirin should not be given to anyone under twenty due to Reye's syndrome). Cough medicine should not be taken. Coughs that are productive, i.e., generate mucus, are the body's way of ridding itself of infection. The mucus should be spat out, not swallowed. Expectorants such as guaifenesin (marketed as Mucinex) and eucalyptus leaf teas can help make coughs more productive.

### Preventing Pneumonia

There is a pneumonia vaccine that can protect children and adults against specific strains of viral and bacterial pneumonia. The vaccine doesn't prevent all types of pneumonia, but it can prevent some of the worst parts of the disease. Children should get pneumococcal vaccines routinely, and older adults, smokers, and those with long-term illnesses should also get vaccinated.

## Bronchitis

Bronchitis is an inflammation of the bronchial tubes that carry air to and from the lungs. It is often accompanied by a cough that produces thick, discolored mucus. Acute bronchitis is usually the result of a cold or virus and improves on its own within a few days, although the cough can linger for weeks.

### *Treating Acute Bronchitis*

Contrary to popular belief, antibiotics are not automatically needed for bronchitis. In fact, 90 percent of bronchitis cases are due to viral infections. Antibiotics are not effective against viruses and should not be used, because they can create antibiotic resistance.

For acute bronchitis, as in pneumonia, do not suppress the cough. Productive coughs help to clear the mucus from airways, reducing infection and making it easier to breathe. Drinking plenty of fluids to help thin the mucus and taking mucolytic drugs to thin and loosen the mucus in airways can make coughs more productive. Using a humidifier at night, especially in a cool, dry climate, can make it easier to breathe and speed healing. But make sure to keep the humidifier clean, because dirty humidifiers can cause respiratory infections by harboring germs.

### *Chronic Bronchitis*

Chronic bronchitis, however, is more severe. Patients have a productive cough that lasts for three months or more, sometimes accompanied by wheezing and shortness of breath. It reoccurs because the bronchial tubes are constantly irritated or inflamed. Smoking is often a cause of chronic bronchitis. Smokers should quit and avoid other respiratory irritants, such as environmental pollutants. The pneumonia vaccine is also helpful.

## HEART TROUBLE

As the strongest muscle in the human body, the heart plays the critical role of pumping blood with its oxygen and nutrients throughout the body. The human heart has four chambers, two atria (upper chambers) and two ventricles (lower chambers). Blood that is low in oxygen is pumped into the right atrium (upper chamber), next into the right ventricle (lower chamber), and then it is then pumped to the lungs to be oxygenated before going to the left atrium (upper chamber), then into the left ventricle (lower chamber), and then it's pumped out through the entire body. Normally, the heart performs this job nonstop at roughly 4,800 beat per hour (115,200 beats per day) without fail. But sometimes, things go wrong.

## Heart Palpitations

When the heart is beating too hard, too fast, or skipping beats, the accompanying feelings are heart palpitations. They can feel like a fluttering in the chest or like the chest is pounding as though running hard and fast even when stationary. In the vast majority of cases, heart palpitations are harmless. If they're infrequent and brief, they don't require medical attention. Relatively benign heart palpitations that don't indicate a heart problem can be triggered by stress, too much caffeine, and even dehydration.

If palpitations are frequent, accompany a history of heart disease, or the palpitations get worse, see a doctor who may conduct some heart-monitoring tests to see if there's a more serious underlying problem, such as an issue with the heart or a thyroid condition. Similarly, if heart palpitations are accompanied by chest pain or discomfort, severe shortness of breath, dizziness, or loss of consciousness, seek immediate emergency medical treatment. These palpitations can be a sign of a much more serious underlying condition that can result in death if left untreated.

## High Blood Pressure

Blood pressure is measured in millimeters of mercury (mm Hg) based on how much blood pressure it takes to raise the mercury 1mm in a mercury manometer. Modern devices range from digital to pressure-based gauges, no mercury necessary, but the measurement has stuck.

Normal blood pressure for an adult is less than 120 mm HG systolic pressure (the upper number that represents the pressure inside the artery as the heart contracts and pumps blood throughout the body) and less than 80 mm HG (the lower number that represents the pressure on the arteries' walls when the heart is at rest). Anything over 140 mm HG for systolic pressure (top) or 90 mm HG for diastolic pressure (bottom) is considered too high. The medical name for high blood pressure is hypertension. While it's possible for blood pressure to dip too low, its severity is based on the suddenness of the dip and whether or not it's causing health problems as opposed to a strict cut off. High blood pressure predisposes one to a number of health conditions, most notably stroke. It can be controlled with a mix of diet, exercise, and medication.

## Hypertrophic Cardiomyopathy

Hypertrophic cardiomyopathy is an abnormal thickening of the heart muscle that makes it more difficult for the heart to pump blood. It's frequently undiagnosed, because many sufferers are asymptomatic. For some people it can lead to chest pain, shortness of breath, and electrical problems with the heart. Roughly one out of every five hundred people is diagnosed with hypertrophic cardiomyopathy, and there's a strong genetic component, so it tends to run in families. Tests to diagnose the condition include echocardiograms that take images of the heart, electro-cardiograms that measure electrical impulses from the heart, and a tread-mill stress test. Treatment generally includes drugs to relieve symptoms and prevent sudden cardiac death; these include blood thinners as well as medications that relax the heart muscle and slow heart rate so that the heart may pump blood more efficiently.

## High Cholesterol

Cholesterol is a fatty molecule that's present in the blood. The body needs cholesterol; it helps break down key nutrients like vitamin D. Issues arise when there's too much cholesterol circulating in the blood stream. High cholesterol predisposes a person to heart disease and heart attacks. There are four cholesterol levels that one should be aware of: total cholesterol, LDL ("bad" cholesterol), HDL ("good" cholesterol), and triglycerides. While total cholesterol should be below 200 mg/dL, the ratio of good cholesterol to bad cholesterol is equally as important. An optimal ratio of good to bad cholesterol is 3.5:1. While age, gender, and genes all affect one's cholesterol levels, diet, weight, and physical activity also affect cho-lesterol level. To prevent high cholesterol, one's diet should be rich in fruits and vegetables while also limiting the amount of saturated fats. Exercise a minimum of three times a week. Weight should remain within a healthy body mass index (BMI) based on weight and height.

## Heart Attack

A heart attack happens when blood flow to the heart is blocked and the heart no longer receives oxygen. The blockage must be cleared quickly or else the part of the heart that is fed by the blocked artery begins to die; then scar tissue forms to replace healthy tissue, which can cause long-lasting problems. If the blockage is severe enough, the person can die.

Symptoms of a heart attack include chest pain or discomfort beginning in the center of left side of the chest and presenting like pressure, squeezing fullness, or pain. Alternatively, it can feel like indigestion. For some peo-ple, the only symptom may be shortness of breath, which can occur on its own or with the chest pain and discomfort. Additional symptoms include discomfort in the jaw, neck, back, upper stomach, or arms; cold sweat; feeling unusually tired for days, without reason; and light-headedness or sudden dizziness. Women in particular are likely to present with atypical symptoms of a heart attack such as light-headedness or tiredness.

If you think you're having a heart attack, you should take an aspirin, which thins the blood, making it easier for blood to get past the blockage and for your heart to pump the blood. Aspirin, however, isn't a curative: it merely buys you a very small amount of time. You still need seek immediate medical attention; surgery is frequently required to remove the blockage.

At the same time, it's important to recognize that heart disease is preventable. Quitting smoking, exercising by walking as little as thirty minutes a day, and eating a heart-friendly diet that's low in processed meats and simple sugars and filled with a diverse array of vegetables all help to reduce the risk of heart disease and heart attack.

## STROKE

While a heart attack is a blockage of blood in the arteries that lead to the heart, a stroke is a blockage of blood in arteries that lead to the brain. Absent oxygen, the cells in a brain start to die within minutes. Left untreated, the patient dies shortly afterward. Strokes are the fourth leading cause of death in the United States.

The two main kinds of strokes are ischemic strokes, which are caused by blood clots, and hemorrhagic strokes, which occur when arteries in the brain leak blood or rupture. A third condition, called transient ischemic attack (TIA) or "mini-strokes," occurs when blood flow to the brain is temporarily interrupted. Brain cells are not permanently damaged, but people with TIA are far more likely to have full strokes.

Symptoms of a stroke occur in the parts of the body controlled by the parts of the brain that are dying. These symptoms include sudden weakness, paralysis or numbness of the face, arms, or legs, trouble speaking or trouble understanding speech, and trouble seeing. There is no way of treating a stroke at home—immediately seek emergency medical care.

### Treating Strokes

Ischemic strokes are treated with drugs to break down clots and prevent further ones from forming. Both aspirin and injections of drugs called tissue plasminogen activators (TPAs) are effective at dissolving clots, but TPAs have to be injected within the first four and a half hours of experiencing stroke symptoms. Surgeons may do surgery to open the artery and remove any plaque that may be blocking it. Alternatively, they may do an angioplasty: a procedure during which a balloon is inserted and inflated in the artery via a catheter to open up the blood vessel. They may also insert a mesh tube into the opening in order to stabilize the artery.

Since hemorrhagic strokes are caused by bleeding in the brain, taking aspirin would NOT be helpful as aspirin is a blood thinner that encourages bleeding. Generally, treatment begins with drugs to reduce pressure in the brain and prevent sudden constrictions. Surgery is used to repair any problems with blood vessels that caused the stroke.

## Preventing Strokes

In both main types of strokes, prevention involves many of the same mechanisms for preventing a heart attack. Patients should maintain a healthy weight by eating diets rich in fruits and vegetables and exercising regularly. If patients have diabetes or high blood pressure, they should keep both under control. Smokers should quit smoking, and it is best to limit the consumption of alcohol. Finally, treat any underlying sleep issues.

## PAIN RELIEF OPTIONS

There are a lot of words that can be used to describe pain: throbbing, pulsing, tingling, aching, pinching, stabbing, and shooting. At its core, pain is nothing more than a sensation that hurts. Whether you stub your toe or cut off your foot, the sensation you are feeling is pain. Acute pain is frequently short-lived but intense. Once the injury goes away, or at least begins to heal, so does the pain. Chronic pain by contrast, may be less painful but constant or frequently reoccurring, like the pain that comes with arthritis.

Dealing with pain depends both on the type of pain—acute versus chronic—and the source of the pain itself. Personal tolerance for pain also pays a key role. While the mechanisms by which the human body experiences pain are well known, pain relief is less well understood. Similarly, some people have higher and lower thresholds for pain. A bee sting may rate a "ten" on the pain scale for one person, while another person may view a broken arm as merely a "two." Pain management is not a one-size-fits-all problem.

# Natural Pain Relief
## Breathing

Breathing can be especially helpful for the sudden onset of acute pain, like with minor injuries. Take deep, slow, controlled breaths that reach all the way down to the stomach when breathing in; the stomach should fully contract when breathing out. Counting to ten is one way to ensure measured breathing. The reason behind this strategy isn't fully understood, but one theory suggests slow breathing dampens the sympathetic nervous system, which controls blood flow and skin temperature. Studies have shown that dampening the sympathetic nervous system dulls pain.

## Meditation

Mindfulness meditation is particularly helpful with managing chronic pain. At least one study has shown that mindfulness meditation can reduce perception of pain by 57 percent. Mindfulness meditation comes in a several forms, but it's generally focused on bring awareness fully to the present moment. Focus on breathing for twenty minutes, merely paying attention to the way that breath moves in and out of the body. Or, focus on breathing in and out as the mind wanders, redirecting it to breathing. Unlike medication, meditation is not a quick fix; it's a practice. But as little as twenty minutes daily can yield tremendous results, not only in pain management but also in reduced stress levels and increased sense of happiness and wellbeing.

## Ice

Ice is nature's anti-inflammatory, both dulling pain and helping to reduce swelling after muscle sprains, tears, or general soreness. The preferred method of treating sprains used to be RICE (rest, ice, compression, and elevation), but studies are increasingly showing that both the rest and ice aspects can actually delay healing of mild to moderate soft tissue injuries. Increasingly, medical practitioners are encouraging people to take part in moderate levels of activity after an injury. They are also limiting use of ice to immediately after an injury, to soothe muscles after using them, or when pain reoccurs. Ice should never be applied directly to the skin.

Instead, wrap the ice in a thin cloth, because ice directly applied can stick to open wounds and cause frostbite. Finally, ice should not be applied for longer than twenty minutes at a time.

### Hot Compress

Heat opens up blood vessels and increases blood flow, which brings oxygen and nutrients that reduce pain in the joints. It also helps to relax sore muscles, ligaments, and tendons. It's incredibly helpful for dealing with stiff joints and chronic muscle and joint pain. Wet heat—a heating pad that has been dampened, a sauna, etc.—are generally thought to be more penetrating than dry heat. Note: most electric heating pads should not get wet. Popular options for heat therapy include hot water bottles, gel packs, electric heating packs, and even a nice hot bath. If using a heat pack, it should not be applied directly to skin (you risk burning the skin). The heat source should be wrapped in a thin towel.

### Massage

Massage is the rubbing and kneading of muscles and joints of the body with hands to reduce tension and pain, a practice that dates back at least three thousand years. In one study, Americans rated massage to be as effective as medication for chronic pain relief. While the traditional image of massage is of someone lying flat on a table while a masseuse gently but firmly strokes the skin, there are a number of massage techniques, including deep tissue massage, that are less relaxing but more therapeutic. And, depending on the site of the pain, massaging one's self is a distinct possibility. Muscle and tendon issues in the legs and feet, for example, are particularly adept at self-care. For most kind of muscular pain, find the knot or trigger point near the site of pain and push on it directly (for ten to one hundred seconds) or try applying a kneading motion using small circular strokes. In terms of intensity, it should be between a four and a seven on a personal pain scale—not a ten! Over time you'll figure out what works best for the injury.

## Pain-Relieving Drugs

### Acetaminophen

Acetaminophen (a.k.a. paracetamol) has been a go-to pain reliever since the 1950s because it doesn't impact stomach lining the way other drugs can. It seems to work by impacting the parts of the brain that receive the body's pain messages and regulate temperature. In recent years, however, acetaminophen has been found to be more dangerous than previously believed. It can become toxic at relatively low levels of consumption, resulting in liver failure, so adhere closely to the dosage instructions. Further, alcohol consumption makes acetaminophen more toxic, so one should not consume it when he or she has been drinking. Lastly, despite the fact that it is widely prescribe for chronic back and arthritis pain, a recent study has found that in a clinical setting it performed no better than a placebo.

## NSAIDs

Non-steroidal anti-inflammatory drugs, better known as NSAIDs, are a class of fever and pain relievers that work by reducing the levels of a hormone-like substance called prostaglandins that triggers the sensation of pain by irritating nerve endings. In addition to reducing pain, these drugs also reduce inflammation, making them particularly useful when pain involves soft tissue and muscles. Unfortunately, they can cause irritation to the stomach lining. Common NSAIDs include aspirin, naproxen, and ibuprofen.

### Aspirin

Also known by the chemical name acetylsalicylic acid, aspirin is used for a wide variety of pain problems. Its use dates back more than two millennia, when pain relievers were originally brewed from the bark of a willow tree. Note: aspirin should not be given to children under the age of eighteen because it can cause Reye's Syndrome, a rapid onset of brain swelling. Aspirin also increases the risk of stomach bleeding and bleeding strokes, but low doses of aspirin can reduce the risk of heart attack among those who are susceptible or have had a previous heart attack. If someone may be experiencing a heart attack, the patient can take aspirin as a form of protection until receiving proper medical attention.

### Naproxen

Also known as Aleve, naproxen and naproxen sodium are commonly used for a wide variety of pain problems. Naproxen has a higher risk of stomach ulcers than ibuprofen, but it has a lower risk of causing complications among those at risk for cardiovascular events like heart attack or stroke.

### Ibuprofen

Often marketed as Advil or Motrin, ibuprofen is commonly used for inflammation, headache, toothache, back pain, menstrual pain, arthritis, and minor injuries. It also has a blood thinning effect, but not as strong as that of aspirin.

### Opioids (Opiates)

Opioids are a group of pain-relieving alkaloid compounds that are either found naturally in the opium poppy plant (codeine and morphine), or created synthetically (oxycodone). Opioids work both by reducing the intensity of the pain signals that reach the brain and affecting the areas of the brain controlling emotion, thus reducing the impact of a painful stimulus. While morphine is almost exclusively used in a hospital setting before and after surgery to reduce severe pain, the rest are prescribed for a wide number of pain-related problems ranging from dental surgery to back pain. Because of the manner in which opioids impact the brain, they can be extremely addictive and rife for abuse. They are not available without a prescription.

### Caffeine

Caffeine, as found in coffee and teas, is a stimulant that affects the nervous system. When added to other pain relievers, caffeine can have a small but perceptible improvement in their pain reduction capabilities. This has been found to be especially true when dealing with headache and joint pains. Excedrin is an example of a combination drug made of acetaminophen and caffeine.

## PREGNANCY AND ITS COMPLICATIONS

Medical improvements over the past one hundred years have transformed reproduction into a routine event, but this wasn't always the case. In the United States in 2013, 18.5 maternal deaths occurred for every 100,000 live births. A century ago it was six hundred per 100,000 births. That said, the risks of childbirth haven't gone away; blood loss and infection are all very real. Preparation for childbirth is still extremely important. Where will you be delivering the baby? Who will help you deliver the baby? What kind of training and certification will they have? What is your contingency plan if things go wrong? What kind of preparation will you be taking to prepare for the process of childbirth? What kind of pain management options will you be considering?

## Labor and Delivery

Labor is the first part of childbirth preceding delivery. Throughout pregnancy and in the weeks leading up to delivery, many women—especially first time mothers—experience false labor, also known as practice contractions or Braxton-Hicks contractions; these are the body's way of preparing for pregnancy and birth. They're different from labor contractions because they tend to be infrequent. Similarly, women may experience a mucus discharge that is reddish or brownish in color. The discharge is most likely the mucus plug that blocks the cervix. Its dissipation means that labor is coming, but it can begin immediately or still be days away

The labor process starts when contractions begin and continue at regular, decreasing intervals. Many women also speak of lower back pain that doesn't go away. And there is the classic breaking of the water. Contrary to its portrayal on TV, it isn't always a gush; it can be a continuous trickle.

### Labor

Labor lasts between twelve to nineteen hours. It begins with the onset of contractions and ends when the cervix is fully open or dilated at roughly ten centimeters. Once contractions begin, monitor the interval between contractions, and keep your doctor up to date on your progression. If you're planning on going to a hospital or birthing center to deliver, the early part of labor can occur at home—just keep yourself comfortable. Your doctor or midwife will tell you when the contractions are frequent enough for you to head to the hospital or birthing center.

Once at the hospital or center, your medical practitioner will monitor your progress, along with the baby's position and wellbeing. The baby should be facing head down toward the pelvis. If the baby is faced the other way with the behind toward the pelvis (a position known as breech), a C-section will most likely be prescribed, as a breeched delivery poses significant risks to both mother and child.

Contractions will grow stronger and tips on breathing and relaxation will come into play until ready to push. The doctor may place a fetal heart monitor to watch your baby's heart rate by placing two straps on your stomach. Then, there will be a transition period where the contractions arrive fast and strong and where you will have little relaxation time. It is at this stage where your cervix is likely fully dilated and the baby is ready to arrive.

## Delivery

This is the stage where the mother starts pushing. On average, it lasts for a span of twenty minutes to two hours. There are a number of birthing positions: squatting, sitting, kneeling, or lying on the back. While some evidence suggests upright positions make delivery easier, comfort is the biggest priority: pick the position that is most comfortable to you. Eventually the baby's head crowns, a final push or two allows him or her to emerge from the uterus, and the medical practitioner cuts the umbilical cord.

## Delivery of the Placenta

Between five and thirty minutes after delivery you'll experience another set of contractions. The placenta, which nurtured the baby throughout its development, will emerge. Occasionally the placenta doesn't come out; this is known as a retained placenta. Lightly tugging on the part of the umbilical cord still attached to the mother may help the placental come out. Otherwise an injection of an obstetric combination drug that causes the womb to contract strongly eases the delivery of the placenta. If it still doesn't come out, then a doctor may need to reach in and remove it by hand, generally using a regional anesthetic to ease any discomfort.

Labor and delivery is an intense experience. Done well, both mother and baby can emerge happy and healthy.

## Rh Factor

Rhesus (Rh) is a type of protein on the surface of blood cells that cause a response from the immune system. Most people are Rh positive. But if a woman who is Rh negative carries an Rh-positive baby (as is common), her immune system may try to create antibodies that attack her baby's blood. An Rh immune globulin shot works to stop the body from developing those antibodies. A shot of Rh immune globulin is also administered to Rh negative women after birth to prevent problems in future pregnancies.

# Spontaneous Abortion

A spontaneous abortion, better known as a miscarriage, occurs when a fetus or embryo dies fewer than twenty weeks after conception. Approximately, 10 to 25 percent of confirmed pregnancies will end in a miscarriage. The percentage of miscarriages is likely higher, because early miscarriages that occur before a woman knows she is pregnant are often mistaken for the menstrual period. A miscarriage does not mean that a woman will be unable to conceive normally moving forward.

A woman can tell that she is miscarrying if vaginal bleeding fills more than one super-size sanitary pad in an hour for two hours in a row. The earlier a woman is in her pregnancy, especially during the first trimester, the more likely it is that the body will complete the miscarriage on its own without the need for medical intervention. The primary treatment under this circumstance is emotional support, since a miscarriage can be emotionally traumatic.

However, sudden chills or fever can be a sign that materials of the pregnancy have remained inside of the woman's body (a septic or infected spontaneous miscarriage), in which case any remaining pregnancy-related tissue must be removed, usually using a process called dilation and curettage. A doctor will widen the cervix and scrape the uterine lining, called the endometrium. The procedure is not particularly comfortable, so it is usually done under general anesthesia to reduce discomfort. Alternatively, a medication like misoprostol can be prescribed to help the body if the miscarriage happens later in the pregnancy. The doctor may also prescribe antibiotics.

## Ectopic Pregnancy

Ectopic pregnancies occur when a fertilized egg implants somewhere other than the uterus, most commonly in the fallopian tube. The pregnancy can't proceed normally, the fertilized egg can't survive, and if it isn't treated, the egg will continue growing and destroy maternal structures. Extreme outcomes include life-threatening blood loss and even death. Ectopic pregnancies are the most common cause of maternal death in the first trimester.

An ectopic pregnancy will register as pregnant on a pregnancy test. The initial indication that something is awry includes light vaginal bleeding with abdominal or pelvic pain, sometimes accompanied by shoulder pain or an urge to evacuate ones bowels. Should the fallopian tube rupture, it will often be accompanied by heavy bleeding inside the abdomen, lightheadedness, fainting, and shock. Ectopic pregnancies are typically diagnosed within the first four to five weeks using either a pelvic exam, an ultrasound, or through blood tests. They're treated either surgically or with shots of the drug methotrexate to stop cell growth and dissolve existing cells. While relatively rare—only 1 to 2 percent of pregnancies are ectopic—women who smoke and those who have had ectopic pregnancies in the past, have a history of pelvic infections or infertility, and women with increased maternal risk are more likely to have an ectopic pregnancy.

# INDEX

Earwax, 133
Eating utensils, 17–18
Ectopic pregnancy, 188–189
Emergency. *See* Medical emergency
EpiPen, 19, 64–65
E-reader, 6
Eye injury, 123–130
Eye irritants, 125–126
Eye patches, 125
Eye rinse, 126

**F**

Feminine care, 12
Fever, 158
Feverfew, 46–47
Filling, tooth, 136
Filtering, water, 31. *See also* Water
    purification
Fire ants, 54–55, 77–78
Fire starting, 16–17, 18,
    36–39
First aid. *See also* Injury; Medical
    emergency
    anaphylactic shock, 61–65
    condoms in, 15–16
    splint in, 39–42
    tourniquet in, 42–44
Fishhook wounds, 117
Flash drive, 6
Flashlights, in bug-out bag, 7
Flotation, condoms for, 17
Flu remedies, 49–51, 157–158
Food
    in bug-out bag, 6–7
    dehydration, 35–36
    refrigeration, 35
    storage, 15, 35

Foot, immersion, 93–94
Foreign bodies
    in ear, 133
    in eye, 126
    in nose, 131–132
Fracture, 131, 143–144
Frostbite, 93
Frostnip, 92

**G**

Gallbladder, 139–140
Gas (digestive), 137
Gauze, 9, 120
Gila monster, 70
Ginger, 48–49
Glasses, 14
Gloves, sterile medical, 8
Glue, skin, 119
Gonorrhea, 154
Granular calcium hypochlorite,
    33–34
Gratitude, 160–161
Gum problems, 135–136

**H**

Headache remedies, 45–47
Heart attack, 179–180
Heart palpitations, 177–178
Heart trouble, 177–180
Heat, 95–97
Heat cramps, 96
Heat exhaustion, 96
Heat stroke, 97
Hemlock, 82–83
Hepatitis B, 154
Hernia, 159
Herpes, 154–155